Sexuality in Mid-Life

Sexuality in Mid-Life

Stephen B. Levine, M.D.

Center for Marital and Sexual Health
Beachwood, Ohio
and Case Western Reserve University School of Medicine
Cleveland, Ohio

Plenum Press • New York and London

Library of Congress Cataloging-in-Publication Data

On file

ISBN 0-306-48446-3 (PB)
ISBN 0-306-45742-3 (HC)

© 1998 Plenum Press, New York
A Division of Plenum Publishing Corporation
233 Spring Street, New York, N.Y. 10013

http://www.plenum.com

10 9 8 7 6 5 4 3 2 1

Printed in the United States of America

To my family for teaching me about love

Preface

I wrote *Sexuality in Mid-Life* to assist clinicians in considering love, sex, intimacy, and dysfunction as they occur in this epoch of the life cycle. The chapters reflect my belief that understanding the processes of living is vital for both the therapist and the patient. Despite my preoccupation with creating a cohesive book, I often thought of these 11 chapters as essays because in this prose form it is traditional for the author to be palpably present in the text. I tried not to hide behind the passive constructions of typical psychiatric books. I wanted to create a book that did not restrict itself to scientific findings, clinical experiences, or ideological traditions. I wanted to discuss relevant issues that were generally avoided by professionals. In approaching the topics of love, extramarital affairs, and menopause, for instance, I hoped to emphasize the developmental potentials inherent in both mid-life's smooth sailing and its underappreciated adversities.

Sexuality in Mid-Life is my third solo-authored book. During the writing of the first two, I thought I was painting a picture of the life cycle of sexuality. When a young woman said something complimentary to me about *Sex Is Not Simple* and quickly added that I had left out any consideration of the sexuality of pregnancy, I was stunned by my oversight. Shortly after *Sexual Life: A Clinician's Guide* was published, I again was taken aback when a middle-aged friend remarked that I did not have much to say about menopause. The awareness that I still possessed life-cycle blind spots proved to be a humbling interruption of my private celebration of the second book. Now that this book is completed, I am a bit anxious about what I omitted.

So much about human sexuality has been collected through clinical experience. So little has been collected through clinical scientific studies. Most of the rigorous studies of sexual topics emanate from psychology professors using their students to measure some topic. These often valuable studies illuminate matters quite different than middle-age developmental possibilities and problems. As most clinicians who have delved a bit into the scientific method know, the accumulations of scientifically derived data and of clinically derived impressions provide no absolute guarantee that the observations are correct. One can easily mismeasure or misperceive a phenomenon very many times. Scientists, clinicians, and authors have good reason to remain tentative about their knowledge and understanding.

My work as a therapist occurs within a group practice where I am surrounded by colleagues with ideas. To each of them I offer my gratitude for their presence, support, and challenges. Stanley Althof, Ph.D., and Candace Risen, L.I.S.W., have been so much a part of my intellectual milieu for over 20 years that it is difficult to discern to what extent my ideas are actually my own. I also want to express my appreciation to Mariclaire Cloutier at Plenum who has continued to be interested in the development of my thinking and who has skillfully assisted me in focusing my ideas.

My largest debt of gratitude, however, remains to my wife, Lillian, whose quiet support, indulgence, sensibilities, and editorial eye have enabled *Sexuality in Mid-Life* to reach the world of readers.

Contents

Sexuality in Mid-Life

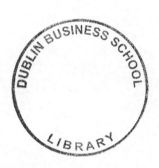

What Is the Nature of Love?

The good life is one inspired by love and guided by knowledge.
—Bertrand Russell[1]

A PSYCHIATRIST CONFRONTS LOVE

The time-honored role of the mental health professions is to take clinical responsibility for the wide variety of problematic emotional states. The distinct focus of this obligation is the relief of emotional suffering, the relief of what our professions more formally call *psychopathology*. To the extent that our work is scientific, it is based on studies of the biological, social, and psychological variables that create, maintain, or relieve these problems. The profound seriousness of psychiatry has not wavered much during this century. However, the patterns of mental anguish that are of greatest interest, ideas about their origins, and how mental health professionals actually function continue to evolve.

How best to prepare mental health professionals for their responsibilities is not as clear. I consider an understanding of the nature of adult love to be one of the proper foundations for work in this field. Although many others might agree, most training programs, in fact, ignore the topic. Three intertwined obstacles keep this subject far from our educational sensibilities. The first is that psychopathology, not health, drives the engine of psychiatry's teaching and research. The processes and possibilities of adult development—that is, concepts of opportunity, ability, conflict, struggle, and mastery or failure—are not the focus of concern of government-funded research, the pharmaceutical industry, clinical training programs, or mental health care delivery systems. In these places, a narrower focus reigns: the investigation and treatment of various states of psychopathology. Mental disorders—psychosis, depression, anxiety, and substance abuse, to name a few—drive the engines.

The second obstacle is that love sounds too trivial for mental health professionals. Love has ubiquitous representations in our culture, from rock-and-roll to soap operas, from low-brow to high-brow art forms. The recurrent message of many of these activities is predictably akin to "All we need is love," a phrase that may work in the theater, the pulpit, or songwriting, but not in the rooms where complex clinical realities are routinely confronted.

The third is that most aspects of love are beyond the research tools of psychology and clinical science and even beyond the less data-bound subjective processes of psychoanalysis and psychotherapy.[2] Science rests on its power to predict outcome. The course of love over the life cycle is widely reputed to be unpredictable. The forces that shape love interact within the privacy of individual subjectivity, where science has never established a firm foothold.[3] Love, however relevant to psychopathology, is too soft a subject for a profession that advertises its base as scientific. As a result, when professionals want to learn about love, we do not immediately think to review some scientific literature.[4] We are more likely to read a novel or short story.[5]

These obstacles no longer deter me from the subject. In 25 years as a clinical psychiatrist, I have learned that the work always pushes me beyond the reach of science into the realm of the patient's subjectivity. I now realize that science is not the only legitimate means of increasing our fund of knowledge or improving our clinical work, it is just the most respected in the larger medical world.[6]

Essayists on love, whether they be philosophers, theologians, literary critics, social scientists, or psychoanalysts, typically prepare their readers for the limitations of their work by commenting on how broad and deep the topic is. They point out that adult love is only one of many types of love that shape and color our lives.[7] They emphasize that multiple viewpoints on love are forever required as no one field, perspective, or person can have the last word on its evolving nature.[8] I echo this standard prelude.

Although I prefer to consider what follows to be a psychiatric perspective, it is misleading to wrap my ideas within the mantle of a profession that has largely avoided the topic. To be fair, I warn you that my thinking about love has been informed by three forces: my practice as a clinician, my individual life experiences in the sphere of love, and my reading.

THE BASIC QUESTION

The subject of this chapter is the type of adult love that aspires to create a sexualized bond that evolves throughout the life cycle. The most basic question is, "What is the nature of this love?" Is its essence a feeling, a force, a figment of imagination, a fixture of culture, a life process, a genetic imperative, or a shared individual and cultural illusion? The philosophy professor Irving Singer, who examined the basic question in great detail, wrote that "the meaning of love is to be found in our propensity to create ideals that liberate us from reality."[9] I am greatly taken with the wisdom compacted into these words, but I think more prosaically. I consider adult love to be, in essence, a powerful ambition—one that is synthesized by four largely unseen phenomena:

1. Long-existent cultural ideals[10]
2. Residues of relationships that begin in childhood
3. Biological systems
4. A person's practical social assessment of the partner

Ideas about love's nature are not the same as definitions; we seek to approach love's essence.

ADULT LOVE IS LARGELY AN IDEAL

Individuals long to live close to their personal ideal form of love. We expend much energy striving to attain harmony in our relationships. Conventionally, this involves mutual respect, behavioral reliability, enjoyment of one another, sexual fidelity, psychological intimacy, sexual pleasure, and a comfortable balance of individuality and couplehood. The latter is a balance between oneness and twoness that creates a sense of sameness out of difference.

Such harmony or the state of ideal love is attainable on earth, but evanescent. Usually, a gap exists between our private sense of ideal love and our actual experience of ourselves and our partner in a relationship. The gap is a source of existential distress and, like all distress, is buffered by an array of competing life demands, defense mechanisms, and self-management techniques. When the buffering system works, one's love, although not continuously or completely harmonious, may be felt as good enough.

THE BEGINNINGS OF LOVE

Falling in Love: One Person

Love stories are thought of as tales about two people. In fact, falling in love requires only one person. Falling in love is an intrapsychic rearrangement process that happens far more often in just one person than in the commonly appreciated two-person situation. One-person love stories are usually experiences of brief mental excitement stimulated by imaginative excursions about what might be, followed by disappointment, embarrassment, and self-castigation about one's foolishness. However, having once fallen, a few people are able to hold onto the idea of another as beloved for a long period of time. For example, a story of one-sided love held in abeyance for a lifetime is compellingly told by Gabriel García Márquez in *Love in the Time of Cholera.*[11] Such stories should not shock experienced psychotherapists, however, because unrequited erotic transferences occur in their patients and can last and last. Others, too, are occasionally aware of those who unilaterally love their co-workers, bosses, neighbors, teachers, or friends. Their singular love may never be perceived by their beloved, may be seen but never acknowledged, or may be cruelly exploited.

Falling in Love: Two People

The well-known two-person phenomenon of falling in love holds an endless charm for us. We repeatedly celebrate it in stories, plays, movies, and gossip. The usual meaning of *falling in love* is the beginning of requited love. Love stories are often about overcoming the initial obstacles to love.

The Defenses

Whether it is a one- or two-person phenomenon, falling in love involves the defenses of denial, idealization and naiveté. They are more or less required during this intrapsychic rearrangement. In the relatively brief process of falling in love, many of those around us feel that we have exaggerated the capacities and minimized the limitations of the newly loved. They often privately say skeptical things to one another about our psychological state including that we are in denial about the obvious capacities and traits of the person; or we are idealizing the new person; we do not appreciate the implications for the future of what we do see.

Throughout the ancient and modern world, new love has the reputation for being transforming.[12] People who fall in love are often keenly aware of the need for something different in their lives. Some think that we fall in love out of this need for psychological or social change. Denial and idealization enable us to break down the boundaries between ourselves and the other to create a new personal identity as a couple. These defenses often convey the deep private hope of personal improvement. "I will be a better person and my life will be better with this person." The skepticism of others also has a voice within us, but it is often quelled by the new psychological intimacy with the partner. Although we may be denying, idealizing, and naive about some aspects of the person, we have a view of the partner that the external skeptics do not have. Some of the perceptions that derive from this knowledge may be more correct and trustworthy than the observations of our friends and family. We hope.

The Central Issues

A developmental issue faces everyone in a new love: Which is correct, my hope-generated judgment or my skepticism? Like other aspects of development, a new love relationship holds much potential, generates new experiences, requires new sensibilities, and will propel the person to a new level of social and psychological existence. But the central personal issue reverberates in the minds of the newly fallen, "Am I being realistic?" A second issue follows on the heels of the first, "Will I be damaged?"

The Emotions

The trepidation that a person feels on entering a new state of love is explained by these central issues, not merely by experience with past relationships.* Calmly dealing with these questions over time is made difficult by the excitement generated by our experiencing the new person as a means of easing some of our important social and psychological burdens. This excitement is variously described as: earthshaking, trancelike, beguiling, or as an amazement, exhilaration, exultation, rapture. Falling in love is often sudden in onset, volcanic in intensity, and sensed as occurring from outside the self, for example, "I was struck by Cupid's arrow." Plato, who mythically considered the basic protohuman form to contain both male and female elements that are separated at birth, explained the array of sensations by having Socrates say that when we fall in love we think that we have finally located our long-missing other half.[13]

Maturation,[14] character style, gender, and culture[15] may modify the process of falling in love somewhat, but the haunting question embedded in this emotional upheaval remains the same: "Am I wise or foolish in pursuing this new relationship?" Although many lovers assume that their new happiness predicts a good future relationship, skeptics, such as Freud, may diagnose a nonpsychotic delusion. Samuel Johnson once quipped that this mental state was a disease best cured by marriage.

An Act of Imagination

If we think of the essential process of falling in love as an act of imagination, we may better understand that terms such as fantasy-driven, illusion, defenses, and affectual stimulation are the ordinary

---

* This is not to say that early life experiences are irrelevant to what we feel and how we behave in this arena. Developmental psychology's basic notions rest on the idea that the quality of early life attachment plays an important unseen role in conduct of early life love affairs.

accompaniments of this momentous mental event. Imagination creates the images of a highly desirable life with a particular person. Something then has to transport the person to the next step. Might we call it faith, risk-taking, or resignation? The attainment of that life becomes the organizing force for much of the person's behavior. Imagination also creates the idealized internal image of the partner that will play a subtle role throughout the life of the relationship. To survive, fresh two-person love must be more than creative imagination, but it may not be less.

Being in Love

Reciprocity between two people is required to create the full intensity of falling in love. An emotional crescendo is reached when we are reassured that something comparable to our internal upheaval over the newly loved is occurring within the other, that is, that we are becoming our beloved's beloved. "Pinch me, am I dreaming? I can't believe it!" A marvelous phase of happiness ensues that we label *being in love*. If falling in love requires a personal act of imagination, then being in love requires the accurate perception of the other's creative burst. Being in love typically lasts much longer than falling in love, but it, too, is not forever. The initial intensity of being in love gradually diminishes and is replaced by a calmer, far less tumultuous period of happiness during which life is increasingly dominated by realistic concerns. Even so, the new partner is experienced as idealized, not merely in the sense that traits are overestimated or failings are not perceived, but in the sense that the person is finally on the way to realizing the grand ambition to love and be loved, and will do everything possible to stay on this high road.

It is here in the uncertain, often-turbulent processes of two people ascertaining whether they are simultaneously in love and resigning themselves to bear the inherent risks, that their willingness to behave sexually often reaches a pinnacle. Whether sexual behavior consists of slow gradual, tentative explorations of each other's bodies or quickly attained genital union, sex is wanted, rehearsed mentally, and experienced with a deliciousness that is long recalled. These early shared sexual pleasures are not only the product of falling in love and being in love, they further enhance the sense of rightness of the union, creating a deepening of the couple's attachment to one another. These psychological and sexual processes are often designated as *passionate love*. Although the term *passionate* conveys the sexual desire inherent in early love, the desire that is passionately stimulated is far more extensive than sexual. It is a desire to be happy, to be understood, to be in agreement about important things, to live an exalted extraordinary life.[16]

The Beginnings of Love Involve More Than the Couple

Falling in love and its happy consequence, being in love, are more than processes occurring between two people. To some extent it is also a subcultural experience. The power, sentimentality, and allure of new love stem from the profound, incompletely knowable hopes that are embedded in the couple. Successfully falling in love restructures life—both psychologically and socially—for the couple, their families, and their friends. Turgenev in his novel, *Spring Torrents,* memorably described the restructuring, "First love is exactly like a revolution: the regular and established order of life is in an instant smashed to fragments; youth stands at the barricade, its bright banner raised high in the air, and sends its ecstatic greetings to the future, whatever it may hold—death or a new life, no matter."[17]

The Hardness of the New Reality

The pleasures of fresh couplehood are relatively quickly challenged by the mundane demands of functioning as a couple. These realities are formidable. A follow-up study of 101 couples who dated exclusively or were engaged, for instance, found that 58% had broken up within 4 years.[18] If new heterosexual couples are able to survive the early tests of their relationship, marriage looms. Marriage adds the complexity of profound commitment to their love that makes their bond far more difficult to dissolve socially, psychologically, morally, economically, and spiritually.

Acting the Role of Being in Love

Western cultures now assume that the emotional excitement of new love is the proper beginning of a relationship. New love is celebrated in songs, movies, and fiction. These model for us what we should feel when we finally find our partner. When people allow the social processes of love to begin even though they are not privately profoundly moved, they may question whether they are "really" in love. "Are my motives for selecting this partner improper?" "Is this relationship a mistake?" "Am I just uncomfortable allowing myself to be emotionally swept away by anything?" As this private dialogue is occurring, many people must act the role of being in love while waiting until they grow to love their partner, just as is said to occur when marriages are arranged. When a relationship fails, our Western assumption about how love ought to begin creates the lamentation "What a fool I was to be involved without love!" However, the intensity of the initial feelings does not protect one from future relationship misery. There is hope for those who managed to marry without the benefit of exultation who did a little acting. No matter if love begins with beguiling charm or diffident practicality, the most enduring challenge is staying in love.

STAYING IN LOVE

The Lofty Purposes

Adult love relationships have a complex implicit purpose: Partners are chosen in the tacit hope that they will accompany, assist, emotionally stabilize, and enrich us as we evolve, mature, and cope with life's other demands. Adult love is expected to combine three elements for each partner as the couple moves through the life cycle: sexual pleasure, cherishing of the person of the partner, and behavioral caring for the partner.

Defenses Are Still Required

To realize these lofty purposes, each of us must rely at times on mechanisms of defense, including idealization, denial, and rationalization. Idealization enables us to hover closer to our ideal of loving and being loved. We idealize our partners in return for their devotion to us; it is an unconscious bargain we make with them: I will continue to bestow love onto you and you will continue to bestow love onto me.

We also need illusions about our partner's capacities, attributes, and attitudes toward us to minimize our disappointment with them. Chief among our illusions is that our partner simply loves us without struggle. We assume this, despite our awareness that it is a recurrent struggle to love our partner. We also routinely rationalize away some of our disappointment by telling ourselves to be *realistic* about what can be expected from any partner. If the reality of our relationships is not close to our ideal, we try to move toward the ideal in the privacy of our minds. And there we may repeatedly emphasize what is close to the ideal—she is a good cook, he is a good father—rather than focus on what is not—I wish she could enjoy sports with me; I wish he were not so asocial. There are good reasons to be so *unrealistic* about our partners: After all, they have been chosen to accompany, assist, stabilize, and enrich us as we grow. Interfering with the long-term processes of love is done at great peril. We should take some hope that some people happily negotiate the years of marriage and attain its final accomplishment—the struggle to love and to be loved is ended. They surrender to the knowledge that they do love in their idiosyncratic ways and so do their imperfect partners. On the way to this distant goal, the internal sense of the partner changes focus many times.

Other Requirements for Managing the Gap

The distress created by the gap between our ideal and the real is far from constant. It ranges from high to low in response to many major and minor external events. Maintaining high-quality psychological and sexual intimacy requires more than defense mechanisms. These dual challenges require good judgment about when to speak and what to say, a commitment to work with good humor toward realizing ideal love, the discipline to allow our loftiest values to govern our lives during the inevitable times of doubt, and the ability to apologize. As we settle into a long-term relationship, we inevitably see our partners more clearly. We see their recurring patterns of behavior, we better realize their strengths and their limitations, and we pass personal judgment on their integrity and trustworthiness. A large part of the private work of being in a relationship is dealing with the disappointment about our partner's styles, capacities, and treatment of us. This work is **not** ordinarily done with the partner; it is done within the self, alone in ongoing dialogues that we have with our disappointed conflicted selves.

Appraisal and Bestowal

Staying in love is the product of two ongoing hidden mental activities: the assessment of the partner's character (appraisal) and the granting of cooperation (bestowal).[19] People often erroneously assume that their partners simply and constantly love them. But a partner notices the other's behavior, interprets it, and decides whether or not to love. When love can be genuinely bestowed, it is typically immediately reflected in cooperation, affection, and enjoyment of the partner. Another important consequence is typically not seen, namely, the shoring up of the idealized internal image of the beloved.

Although we do not love our partners constantly, we allow them to think that we do. They make erroneous assumptions because we do genuinely feel love for them sometimes. And when we do not, our commitment to behave in a kind, helpful fashion may carry the moment. Our idealized image of our partner enables us to act loving because we do feel loving toward the partner's image—if not to the actual partner sulking upstairs. Continuing negative appraisals, however, interfere with sensations we called love, the commitment to love, and the internal image of the partner as lovable. We then find it difficult to bestow affection and cooperation and we cease to enjoy our partners.

Many people seem to expect to be loved regardless of their behavior or capacities. Young children are (ideally) loved unconditionally, older children and siblings are to some extent as well, but it is unlikely that most adults can continue to bestow love without some degree of positive appraisal. For unconditional love, adults usually turn to God.

Privately, many individuals are disappointed in how they actually feel about their partner. Their love feels to them tarnished, inferior, unfortunate because of their negative appraisals. They long to love as they love their infants and young children: a love to die for, one with a reassuring purity and intensity. The love for an infant is not as challenging as staying in love with an adult. When adults use infant-parent love as a model for their love, they are bound to be deeply disappointed.

The Intrapsychic Mental Buffering of Distress

Theoretically, distress about the inescapable gap must be buffered in some way. There must be an adaptive mental balance mechanism in operation under ordinary conditions because the fluctuations of distress can be sudden and dramatic.[20] When some new negative appraisal—such as realizing the social limitations of the spouse—destabilizes the balance, the resulting shift may be manifested by a sudden new pessimistic view of the partner. The person may think: "I am no longer in love. I am no longer willing to work privately to remain in this relationship. I have been kidding myself for too long." The person begins to appraise with a new harsher standard and to rewrite the history of the relationship. Bestowal ceases. Even apparently good relationships prove to be precariously balanced intrapsychically.

When such private destabilization occurs, the person may develop considerable anxiety, panic, guilt, or depression. Many of these intrapsychic dramas pass unnoticed by the spouse and family, or if their effects are noted, their source is not perceived.

LOVE EXISTS IN PRIVACY

We know about the precarious balance of relationships because relationships exist in the deepest privacy of our individual psyches. Dependably affectionate, faithful, well-behaved people frequently express anger, disappointment, and outrage to themselves, and imagine leaving their spouses for an improved version—all in this privacy, the same privacy in which idealization used to occur.

The culture, however, is more familiar with the idea that love and loving relationships are both internal and external to each person. We emphasize that love is something that exists between two parties. When we observe couples being affectionate—that is, when the love that privately exists spills over the boundaries of self and social situations—we conclude that they really love each other. It is safer for mental health professionals to assume that love resides in two persons' psyches—hopefully simultaneously. What they exchange publicly or privately may reflect their continuing ability to enjoy and idealize one another or may conceal their acting the part of love because of private disappointment or resentment. Therapists hear sentences like this from abandoned persons: "We made love just two days before and told each other how much we loved one another." Couples seeking marital therapy frequently comment on the irony that "Everyone thinks we are the best, most loving couple." And, therapists repeatedly encounter an inexpressive spouse who is deeply attached to a partner, but is not able to behaviorally or verbally express it.

What is said and done in a relationship is not as crucial as the partner's interpretation of what is said and done. Behavior works if the partner interprets it as meaning "I am loved; this is simply my partner's way." Of course, this conclusion sometimes is an illusion. The illusion of being loved buffers both the fluctuation of distress between the ideal and the real and the other distresses of everyday life. Here is, once again, Singer's quote: The meaning of love is to be found in our tendency to create ideals that liberate us from reality.

Privacy is an arena where many relevant dramas routinely occur. These include the balancing acts between: appraisal and bestowal; feelings thought of as love and those thought of as aggression; attractions to others and moral constraints; alternative meanings considered for the same spousal behaviors.

As the perception "I am not loved" or the conclusion "I do not love this person" emerges in consciousness and gradually thunders its way into the couple's dialogue, abandonment becomes a distinct possibility. Both partners, their children, and their extended family may then readily earn a DSM-IV label, if a mental health professional is anywhere near them.

HOW WE USE THE WORD LOVE

Here are some synonyms for the verb: *admire, adore, cherish, fancy, idolize, appreciate, enjoy, relish, savor, desire*. There are more synonyms for the noun: *attachment, fondness, sentiment, fancy, shine, passion, ardor, fervor, heart, flame, desire, yearning, worship, accord, devotion, adoration, affection, beloved, benevolence, endearment, friendship, liking*. The same word is used to describe our pleasure in wearing a favorite sweater and our complex synthesis of experience with a spouse of 50 years; we say we love a particular musical group and we label the rush of emotions at our child's wedding ceremony with the same word. It is equally useless to try to delineate a singular meaning for *love* in our language or to assume that terms such as *passionate love, romantic love, true love, pure love, real love, companionate love, limerance, spiritual love, lust, eros,* and *sexual love* have discrete meanings to most of those who use them. Is it a wonder that mental health professionals have not directly entered into this land of the undefined?

Recently, Sternberg has offered a new vocabulary of love.[21] He explains the dominant forms of adult love by drawing a triangle. Its three points are:

- *intimacy,* by which he means friendship
- *passion,* by which he means sexual desire and sexual pleasure
- *commitment,* by which he means the decision to be together

Each element has a different time course, passion being assumed to be the shortest. From these elements he constructs six categories of love:

1. *Infatuation*=passion without commitment or intimacy
2. *Romantic love*=passion and intimacy
3. *Consummate love*=passion, intimacy, and commitment
4. *Companionate love*=intimacy and commitment
5. *Fatuous love*=passion and commitment without intimacy
6. *Empty love*=commitment without intimacy or passion

An adult love relationship is a changing or dynamic phenomenon with a potential to move through many definable points over time. Although these terms can describe a couple's relationship at a particular time, the scientific attempt to model love needs to be viewed with both interest and humor.

"I LOVE MY PARTNER BUT I AM NOT IN LOVE WITH MY PARTNER"

This sentence is frequently uttered by men and women in clinicians' offices and, of course, elsewhere. What could it mean? When I ask patients to explain, the ensuing dialogue usually meanders widely and is peppered with examples to illustrate why the declaration was made. But what does it mean in terms of the concepts that are being discussed in this chapter? Here is my current understanding. It may mean that although the person is still committed to the idea of remaining in the relationship and has fond memories of their life together ("I still love my partner..."), the internal image of the partner as lovable has been erased ("I no longer am in love with my partner"). It also may mean that although I recognize that we have shared so much of our lives together and that my partner is inextricably part of me ("I still love my partner"), I no longer am able to cherish this person or experience the same sense of belonging to one another during sex ("I no longer am in love with my partner"). This may not capture what everyone who utters that sentence is attempting to convey. The sentence may only signify that the person used to experience a more exulted form of love—for instance, consummate love—and now has slipped into a less appealing phase—for instance, empty love. The murkiness of the concept of love and its numerous synonyms makes it difficult to be anything but unhelpfully arbitrary when trying to define adult love. It is easier to suggest what love is not.

LOVE IS NOT SIMPLY A FEELING

Most writers refer to love as an emotion. Here is just one typical example from a recent art book on the subject: "Love is the most complex and important of all human emotions."[22] Tomkins[23] and Nathanson[24] have taken great pains to delineate the nine basic affects. They consider *affects* to be hard-wired neural capacities with which all humans respond in gradient fashion to the environment. Love per se is not one of them. They distinguish the conscious experience of stimulated neural capacity, which they label *feelings*, from *emotions*, which are feelings after they have acquired a personal and cultural context. For example, a child's *feeling* of envy is made into a guilt-tinged *emotion* by learning from his family that envy is a sin. Using the Tomkins/Nathanson scheme, love is not a single feeling; it is an interpretation based on a series of emotions—that is, feelings colored by past experience and associations with each feeling. The emotions that we call love are highly individually defined points on two affective gradients: interest→ excitement and enjoyment→joy.

It is perplexing to find that so many authors refer to love as a basic emotion.[25] Love is an intrapsychic state that is built with an array of considerations and emotions that stem from complex evolving psychological processes such as appraisal, attachment, idealization, hope, sexual experience, and commitment.[26] But the idea that love is a basic emotion is so ingrained in our language, thought, and culture that we probably cannot stop misleading ourselves. Love is far more complicated than sadness, anger, fear, pleasure, pride, or joy.

Gandhi emphasizes that love is not simply a feeling. He says that love is a force in nature—the essence of life—because it brings two separate people together into a new entity. He calls love an ontological force.[27] The clergy routinely use the concept of love with sophistication about its nature. They tend to refer to love as the situation between two consenting persons who are committed to caring for and about another. In the fourth century BC, Plato emphasized that love was the desire and pursuit of the whole.

LOVING THE PARTNER

The natural history of adult love begins with the anxious excitement of falling in love. It soon gives way to a more tranquil pervasive happiness of being in love and eventually evolves into loving the partner. This progression has been referred to as the evolution of passionate love into companionate love.[28] We do not remain in love forever in the being-in-love sense. But we do say to ourselves and to others that we love our partners. The quality, intensity, and frequency of our enjoyment of our partner evolve. Our love, once fresh and filled with possibility, soon becomes the new structure of our lives. As this further unfolds, the sensations that we once interpreted as love may be less obvious to ourselves and others.

Loving the partner is now closer to an attitude forged by commitment to values and personal discipline than to mere emotion. When love begins, emotions dominate; their subtle meanings relate to the possibilities of significantly changed structures of our lives. By the time we are in the loving-the-partner phase, the new structures of our lives predominate; emotions become subtle. Loving the partner rests on our appraisal of the degree to which mutual respect, behavioral reliability, enjoyment of one another, sexual fidelity, psychological intimacy, sexual pleasure, and the balance of individuality and couplehood exist in our relationship. Loving the partner also rests on the strength of the internal idealized image of the partner. Of course, our appraisals and our internal image are related. The emotions of love during this long phase do not usually ascend to predominance unless there is a threat of or actual loss, although we are expected to symbolically acknowledge our love through gift giving at birthdays, anniversaries, and holidays.

LOVE IS A LONG-TERM BATTLE FOR MANY

Adult love is a lofty human potential that often has a disappointing outcome. The United States has the highest divorce rate in the world.[29] Statistics for first and second marriages in the United States suggest that 50% end in divorce. Divorce statistics are thought to underestimate the casualties within long-term relationships because of the many people who stay married despite their disappointments.

Casualties are everywhere. Failures of adult love are major public health problems, both for adults and for children. But, we in the mental health professions are wary to say so, to concentrate on the problem, or to have our professional vocabulary reflect our awareness of the impact of failures in the sphere of love on all of those involved.

Genuineness and Staying in Love

Erich Fromm suggested that long-term love requires the remeeting of two people at their emotional genuineness.[30] This idea of genuineness recurs in various literatures. Some psychoanalysts, for example, understand that over decades, adult love reflects what we face in life, how well we face it, and the degree to which our partners can actually be with us in genuineness. Love is about the battles we fight within ourselves to simply be genuine and how their outcome may change subtly with each engagement.

Overcoming Narcissism and Increasing Devotion to the Partner and Couple

Although ideas alone are insufficient to help many people in relationship difficulty, mental health professionals might begin to conceptualize how to love. My suggestions rest on the ideas that staying in love requires overcoming one's narcissism and increasing one's devotion to the partner and the couple. Accomplishing this increases the ease with which a partner can bestow love. This is not *the* formula for happiness. It leaves out the individual art of balancing the needs of the self and the needs of the couple and all of the complexity created by our individual past experiences. The idea of a formula for relationship happiness is naively presumptuous. Because staying in love is such a developmental challenge and because people deem their relationships as failures for such a wide variety of reasons, mental health professionals can only be students of the subject. I offer these suggestions while understanding the ineffable nature of staying in love.

1. Develop your capacity to simply listen to your partner speak.
2. Make clear to your partner what you like to do in life without demanding anything.
3. Err on the side of putting the good of the couple and the good of the partner ahead of your interests.
4. Give your partner the benefit of the doubt when you feel that you have been mistreated.
5. Speak frequently from the heart about subjects other than personal unhappiness with your partner.
6. Smile about your personal ambitions, knowing that most people do not achieve them.
7. Value sexual behaviors highly, even the inevitable disappointing ones.
8. Be aware that your partner's perception that you are generally interested in satisfying your partner's sexual needs is vital to the growth of love.
9. Love your body and its pleasures; stop taking your bodily imperfections so seriously.
10. Consider that integrity, honesty, and respect breed love, love breeds good sex, and good sex breeds love. It is a feedback loop.

11. Own and express your emotions, but don't always assume that they are the most important aspects of any interpersonal situation.
12. Tell your partner how much you value loving and having sex, and don't be embarrassed to admit that although you are satiable when it comes to sex, you are insatiable when it comes to being loved.
13. Do not abandon your ideal of love just because your partner is currently falling short of meeting its requirements.

LOVE AS A ROAD MAP OF DEVELOPMENT

Tasks of development are the inevitable issues that must be confronted by most individuals as they change. For the vast majority of adults—regardless of gender, orientation, or subculture—finding a life mate and learning how to happily pass through the life cycle together is a crucial developmental task. I view the observations about the three phases of love as a road map for this intrapsychic and interpersonal task. Understanding adult development in this manner is not a theoretical revolution, it may not even be a revelation for some readers. But it may help many mental health professionals to more clearly understand what is being said in their offices.

WHAT IS THE SIGNIFICANCE OF LOVE TO PSYCHIATRY?

Today, two powerful forces continue to keep love on the extreme periphery of psychiatric consciousness. The first is economic. All of the confusing demands of the emerging funding systems are currently driving services in the direction of diagnosis, pharmacotherapy, and brief psychotherapy. The second is ideological, that is, the shift of psychiatry's interest to the biology of our brains from the meaning-making function of our minds.

Love is one important door to understanding both humanity and healing. In case the foregoing has not persuaded you that concepts of love may assist our work with various psychopathologies, I offer six reasons to keep these concepts in our professional dialogue:

1. *Because problems of love are often related to psychiatric diagnoses.* One of our central tasks in life is to "keep it together."[31] Among the high-prevalence, emotionally evocative existential dilemmas that we are required to "keep together" are those that derive from our love lives. When we fail, and lose our capacity to contain and well-manage ourselves, we often qualify for a diagnosis. Our emotional decompensations can be more fully understood and often better treated if clinicians grasp the thwarted ambitions that trigger symptoms. Much of the anguish of ordinary adult lives involves personal and interpersonal impediments to loving and being loved. Psychiatrists can become so preoccupied with properly identifying and medically treating anguish that we lose sight of the possibility that the symptoms may have arisen in response to actual or threatened failures in love. The idea that failure in the sphere of love may lead to profound and lingering states of anguish should be considered by us, however, because helping people often requires making sense of their emotional states and restoring dignity to them about their ambitions.

2. *Because love is what patients talk about.* The absence of love, the fear of love, the mishandling of falling in love, threat of losing love, the inability to gracefully cope with the loss of love are the major themes that are discussed in the doctor–patient dialogue when the doctor allows it to move beyond diagnosis and pharmacotherapy. Other issues are also discussed. But what gets more airtime: work or love? siblings or lovers? the aspiration to be rich or the aspiration to be loved?

3. *Because love is an important factor in emotional and physical health.* Love is widely conceptualized in the literature of various disciplines to promote stability, positive self-regard, emotional growth or maturation, physical health, and longer life. Love is good for the immune system.[32] Loss of love through death or divorce is associated with a variety of psychological and physical difficulties.[33]

4. *Because love is often the subtle ingredient in therapeutic improvement.* In therapies that tolerate discussion of what the patients feel about the therapist, therapists soon learn that affection for, excitement over, and sexual desire for the thera-

pist are routine. Therapists often have to deal with their own affection, excitement over, and sexual desire for the patient. These emotional phenomena even happen in those therapies without an ideological support for them because the trusting intimacy of therapy routinely provokes love and eroticization of the therapist.[34]

5. *Because not understanding love may predispose mental health professionals to ethical violations.* Some of the most egregious ethical violations during the life cycle of mental health professionals of both sexes involve the lack of understanding of and poor capacities to deal with the emotional arousal stimulated within the psychological intimacy of patient care.[35]

6. *Because love is necessary to understand sexual health and dysfunction.* One needs a concept of love to understand the vagaries of sexual desire and sexual function in all persons, even those for whom love is unattainable and those for whom it is antithetical to sexual pleasure.[36]

The Nature of Love, the Subject of Psychiatry

Love, impossible to define because of its individuality and evolution, is a force, a fixture of culture, a product of imagination, an evolving intrapsychic and interpersonal process, an ideal, and a shared individual and cultural illusion. Our patient care might improve if we stopped avoiding the topic and grew skeptical about the common tendency to focus on love as it occurs in the young. The subject of love reminds mental health professionals, regardless of their ideological bent, that clinical work cannot be reduced to mere objectivity nor can it lose sight of its ultimate relevance to the major issues of living. The richness and the failures of the human potential are the business of the mental health professions.

REFERENCES

1. Kuntz, P.G. *Bertrand Russell.* Twayne: Boston, 1986, p. 107.
2. Kernberg, O. *Love Relations: Normal and Pathological.* Yale University Press: New Haven, 1995.

3. Rosenthal, L. *The World Treasury of Love Stories.* Oxford University Press: London, 1995, p. xiv.

4. Liebowitz, M.R. *Chemistry of Love.* Little, Brown: Boston, 1983.

5. Gaylin, W. *Rediscovering Love.* Viking: New York, 1986.

6. Lear, J. *Love and Its Place in Nature: A Philosophical Interpretation of Freudian Psychoanalysis.* Farrar, Straus, & Giroux: New York, 1990.

7. Fehr, B., and Russell, J.A. Concept of love viewed from a prototype perspective. *Journal of Personality and Social Psychology* 60:425–438, 1991.

8. Hatfield, E., and Rapson, R.L. *Love and Sex: Cross-Cultural Perspectives.* Allyn & Bacon: Boston, 1996.

9. Singer, I. *The Nature of Love: 3 The Modern World.* University of Chicago Press: Chicago, 1987, Chapter 10.

10. Singer, I. *The Nature of Love: 1 Plato to Luther.* University of Chicago Press: Chicago, 1965.

11. Márquez, G.G. *Love in the Time of Cholera.* Knopf: New York, 1988.

12. Ackerman, D. *The Natural History of Love.* Random House: New York, 1994.

13. Plato. *The Symposium* (B. Jowett, ed.). Tudor Publishing: New York, 1956, pp. 315–318.

14. Emerson, R.W. Love. *Essays: First and Second Series.* Vintage Books: New York, 1990, pp. 97–107.

15. Fisher, H. The nature and evolution of romantic love. In: W. Jankowiak (ed.), *Romantic Passion: A Universal Experience?* Columbia University Press: New York, 1995, pp. 24–41.

16. Alberoni, F. *Falling in Love: A Revolutionary Way of Thinking about a Universal Experience* (L. Venuti, translator). Random House: New York, 1983.

17. Turgenev, I. *Spring Torrents.* Penguin Books: New York, 1980, p.100.

18. Sprecher, S. Two sides to the breakup of dating relationships. *Personal Relationships* 1:199–222, 1994.

19. Singer, I. *The Nature of Love: 2 Courtly and Romantic.* University of Chicago Press: Chicago, 1984.

20. deRougemont, D. *Love Declared: Essays on the Myths of Love.* Pantheon: New York, 1963.

21. Sternberg, R.J. Triangulating love. In R.J. Sternberg and M.L. Barnes (eds.), *The Psychology of Love.* Yale University Press: New Haven, 1988, pp. 119–138.

22. Tresidder, M. *The Secret Language of Love.* Chronicle Books: San Francisco, 1997.

23. Tomkins, S. *Affect/Imagery/Consciousness—Volume 4: Cognition, Duplication and Transformation of Information.* Springer: New York, 1992.

24. Nathanson, D. *Shame and Pride.* Norton: New York, 1992.

25. Fischer, K.W., Shaver, P.R., and Carnochan, P. How emotions develop and how they organize development. *Cognition and Emotion* 4:81–127, 1990.

26. Jankowiak, W. W. (ed.). *Romantic Passion: A Universal Experience?* Columbia University Press: New York, 1995, p. 4.

27. Walsh, A. *The Science of Love: Understanding Love and Its Effects on Mind and Body.* Prometheus Books: Buffalo, 1991.

28. Hatfield, E., and Rapson, R.L. *Love, Sex, and Intimacy: Their Psychology, Biology, and History.* HarperCollins College Publishers: New York, 1993.

29. Fine, M.A., and Fine, D.R. An examination and evaluation of recent changes in divorce laws in five Western countries: The critical role of values. *Journal of Marriage and the Family* 56:249–263, 1994.

30. Fromm, E. *The Art of Loving: An Inquiry into the Nature of Love.* Harper & Row: New York, 1956.

31. Havens, L. Lecture. 1995 American Psychiatric Association Meeting, Miami.

32. Smith, D.F., and Hokland, M. Love and salutogenesis in late adolescence: A preliminary in-vestigation. *Psychology: A Journal of Human Behavior* 25:44–49, 1988.
33. Stroebe, W., and Stroebe, M.S. *Bereavement and Health: The Psychological and Physical Consequences of Partner Loss*. Cambridge University Press: New York, 1987.
34. Levine, S.B. *Sexual Life: A Clinician's Guide*. Plenum: New York, 1992, Chapter 4.
35. Lazarus, J. Ethical issues in doctor–patient sexual relationships. *Psychiatric Clinics of North America* 18(1): 55–70, 1995.
36. Levine, S.B. On Love. *Journal of Sex & Marital Therapy* 21(3):183–191, 1995.

Psychological Intimacy

Mental health professionals swim in murky waters, sometimes so preoccupied with their therapeutic destinations that they fail to notice that the suspending medium is not actually clear.

Love, intimacy, empathy, sexual desire, maturation—clinicians never seem to have the luxury of using concepts with singular meanings. This is both our strength—we have comfortably adapted to ambiguity—and our weakness—we fail to recognize that our therapeutic destinations are unattainable. In this chapter and the next, for instance, we will try to understand how the processes of love relate to psychological intimacy and sexual desire. The question may ultimately be impossible to clarify because of the fuzziness inherent in each concept. Before this cynical conclusion is reached, however, I want to look at the matter more closely. At the very least, a separate, stand alone understanding of intimacy and desire may be achieved. At best, their intersections can be appreciated.

PSYCHOLOGICAL VERSUS SEXUAL INTIMACY

Intimacy implies contact with our innermost selves. Both *intimate* and *intimacy* may refer to innermost touches that are psychological, physical, or both. Whereas *psychological intimacy* connotes familiarity, understanding, affection, and love, the unmodified term *intimacy* does nicely when one wants to delicately refer to, but not name, sexual behaviors. *Intimacy* also does well to communicate a feeling of closeness. Intimacy of either kind usually implies privacy. Intimacies occur within

25

definable boundaries and are deemed appropriate or inappropriate depending on context. In the vast majority of social contexts, extensive or deep intimacies are avoided; behavior is more polite, functional, and superficial than personally significant or touching.

MENTAL HEALTH PROFESSIONALS SELL PSYCHOLOGICAL INTIMACY FOR A LIVING

We mental health professionals are expected to be able to quickly form psychologically intimate relationships in order to assess, diagnosis, and begin to offer our patients relief from their difficulties. Psychological intimacy is one of our basic tools. In a sense, we earn our livings through one-sided intimacy. It is an easy step for us to understand the more demanding two-sided intimacies that are relevant to both love and sexual desire. As a result of our familiarity with the concept, what follows will seem quite basic to an experienced therapist. These ideas create a foundation to understand the conundrums that grip our patients and ourselves in the spheres of love, sexual behavior, and psychotherapy.

The First Step

Psychological intimacy begins with one person's ability to share her or his inner experiences with another. This deceptively simple-sounding capacity actually rests on three separate abilities:

1. The capacity to know what one feels and thinks
2. The willingness to say it to another
3. The language skill to express the feelings and the ideas with words

An incapacity of any of these limits the chance of establishing and maintaining psychological intimacy. For instance, some people do not recognize what they feel, even when their feelings are intense. The best they can do is to say that they are "upset" before or after they behave in some problematic manner. Others do not trust anyone enough to share their inner experiences. Still others are limited by their language skills;

they know what they are experiencing but they cannot explain it. The crucial first step toward psychological intimacy is the sharing by one person of something from within the inner self. What is shared need not be elegantly said, lofty in its content, or unusual in any way; it just needs to be from the inner experience of the self—from the continual monologue of our self-consciousness, from our subjectivity.

The Second Step

For intimacy to occur, the listener has to respond to the speaker in a manner that conveys:

1. A noncritical acceptance of what is being said
2. An awareness of the importance of the moment to the speaker
3. A grasp of what is being said

It also helps a great deal if the listener feels that it is a privilege to hear what the speaker has to say. We mental health professionals are expected to be excellent listeners, that is, to so well understand these ideas that they are automatically incorporated into our professional activities. We may still have our subtle variations from one mental health professional to another, but generally speaking, when a professional and a patient are in conversation, the patient's lack of self-awareness, unwillingness to share, or inability to express what is felt are expected to be the only obstacles to our shared intimacy.

The common errors of inadequate listeners should not occur in professional conversations. In ordinary social interactions, when a listener negatively judges what is being said by saying, "You shouldn't feel that way!" or doesn't acknowledge the significance of what is being said by impatiently remarking, "Can't this wait? Don't you see how busy I am?" or listens but misses the point of the speaker's words, intimacy will not occur.

THE DEFINITION OF PSYCHOLOGICAL INTIMACY

When the patient and the professional perform their respective tasks reasonably well, psychological intimacy occurs. The two people connect; they share a transient rarefied pleasure. The pleasure has at least several components.

1. The patient's pleasure is in large part solace—a form of peace or contentment that results from sharing the inner self, being listened to with interest, and being comprehended. Solace is the response to being seen, known, understood, and accepted.
2. However, intimacy also brings the sense of excitement, energy, and an uplifting of mood. Overall, the experience of intimacy for the patient may be stunning. This flow of emotion may, in and of itself, immediately offer both hope and relief. This response enables professionals to "sell" psychological intimacy because people in emotional distress need and want the restoration of hope.
3. The professional's pleasure results from hearing about the speaker's inner experiences. The professional is trusted enough to be told, competent enough to have enabled the telling, perceptive enough to accurately summarize the speaker's story, and wise enough to respond with interest without censure. The quieter pleasures of intimacy for the clinician should be far more routine. Clinicians are somewhat jaded by their experience with intimacy. But new clinicians learning our skills are often themselves stunned and excited by what they have facilitated. They, too, feel a new contentment.

Is psychological intimacy merely the transient occurrence in two people of some degree of pleasure—solace, contentment, excitement, or pleasure—as the result of conversation? Yes. The importance of psychological intimacy cannot be immediately understood from its occurrence, however. The moment of intimacy is vital for the processes that it may stimulate.

Two-Sided Intimacy

Intimacy has two basic forms. If the conversation continues with the speaker speaking and the listener listening, it is one-sided, but if they switch roles, the intimacy is two-sided. One-sided psychological intimacies are common between children and their parents, patients and health care professionals, clients and lawyers or accountants, and advice-seekers and clergy. Two-sided intimacies are the basis of friendships, love relationships, and are the best day-in, day-out aphrodisiacs ever discovered. Professional intimacies that begin as one-sided and become two-sided are a recognized danger. This is the path followed by professionals who have sexually exploited their patients.[1]

Within these two basic forms, of course, there are countless degrees of self-disclosure and nuances of attention and understanding. No two intimacies are quite alike; each relationship is uniquely rich or poor in its possibilities. Individuals who have seen two therapists often are aware that each professional, although helpful, makes an important contribution to the different intimate atmosphere that occurs. Psychological intimacy is much written about in lay publications, where it is highly lauded as a readily attainable state between two people. Lay discussions rarely define the term. They do not generally emphasize the inherent uniqueness of intimacies for every dyad. They often do not dwell on the fears provoked by being seen, known, and understood and the widespread defenses against the experience. In these lay publications, the fears and defenses of men are better appreciated than those of women.

SHORT-TERM CONSEQUENCES OF TWO-SIDED PSYCHOLOGICAL INTIMACY

The Bond, Visible and Invisible

On the way to the solace of being understood, and on the way to the pleasure and privilege of hearing another person's inner self, powerful internal processes are stimulated within each speaker/listener. Most outside observers can recognize that the reciprocal sharing of the inner monologue with a person who receives it well creates a bond between the speaker and listener. Thereafter, each regards the other differently. The two people are together in a new way: They glance at each other differently; touch each other differently; laugh together differently; and can continue to readily discuss other aspects of their private selves.

Yet much more occurs within the two people than can be observed from outside of them. Within both the speaker and the listener, there is a feeling of attachment, a loss of the usual social indifference, a vision of the person as special. Intimate conversations ignite new processes. The listener becomes internalized within the speaker and, as both are performing each role, they internalize one another. "She is *my* new friend!" Internalization, the invisible bond, has predictable consequences. These include:

1. Imagining the person when she or he is not present
2. Inventing conversations with the person
3. Preoccupation with the person's physical attributes
4. Anticipation of the next opportunity to be together, that is, missing the person
5. Dreaming about the person
6. Thoughts about that person as a sex partner

The intensity of these consequences varies from relationship to relationship.

All of this may be summarized by simply saying that when two-sided psychological intimacy occurs, we begin to weave the person into our selves. Our new intimate partner is not only reacted to as a unique individual, she or he stimulates thoughts, feelings, and worries that we previously experienced in relationship to others. When this process occurs in a professional one-sided psychotherapeutic intimacy, we designate it *transference*. Sometimes we try to use patients' transferences to us to educate them about their past experiences. Ideally, such therapy helps patients to peel off the transferences to significant others in their lives so that they can react to their partners on their own merits rather than in terms of how others treated them years ago. For our purpose of understanding the consequences of psychological intimacy, however, it is important to realize that transference is our professional term for what occurs in therapy. It is also, however, the ordinary intrapsychic response to two-sided psychological intimacy. This is not generally well conceptualized outside of our field. Outside of therapy, strong transferences are merely perceived as trouble.

A Closer Look at the Sixth Consequence

The amount of time required to imagine the person as a sex partner—that is, the speed of the eroticization provoked by intimacy—is modified by at least seven factors: age; sex; sexual orientation; social status; purpose in talking together; the nature of other emotional commitments; the person's attitudes toward private sexual phenomena. If the pair consists of a comparably aged, socially eligible heterosexual man and woman, the erotization triggered by sharing of some aspects of their inner selves can occur with lightning speed—in both of them. Similarly, for a homosexual pair of men or women, eroticization can occur in a flash. The stimulation of the erotic imagination may never occur, take a long time to occur, or occur only in a fleeting disguised way depending on how these seven factors line up. Many adult psychological intimacies do not lead to eroticization. Friendships are valued because they afford an opportunity to share the self without the intrapsychic burden of eroticization.

We need to be a bit skeptical about certain friendships, however. The specific emotional experiences that occur as a result of intimate conversations are usually guarded with extreme care. They can be exceedingly exciting both generally and erotically. Some individuals who are new to intimate conversations may express fear concerning their intense responses to their new friend. They feel so excited as to wonder if they are losing their minds. The power of the excitement of a new psychological intimacy with a friend is strikingly similar to the power of the imaginative burst of falling in love. Might we speak of falling in love with a friend as a nonromantic form of falling in love? When people recognize that they are falling in love with a potential sexual partner, they at least have the culture's teaching to understand their general and erotic excitement. Some friendships, however, end abruptly without satisfying explanation because one person cannot tolerate the excitement it creates. In response to the private eroticization of the mutually revealing conversations, the individual may worry that the relationship is "homosexual" or could lead to sexual behavior. They may not see that forming a new friendship and falling in love with a potential life partner are qualitatively similar. Although psychological intimacy is generally considered to be a positive process, some individuals are unnerved by their internal responses to it and spend their entire lives aspiring to emotional closeness but subverting it. The usual reply to the frustrated spouse is, "I don't know why I do that."

THE LONG-TERM EFFECTS OF PSYCHOLOGICAL INTIMACY

Without repetition of the solace/pleasure experience, the positive consequences of intimacy may be short-lived. For two-sided psychological intimacy to fully blossom, periodic sharing of aspects of the inner self is required. There are good reasons to continue to share over time. Re-attaining psychological intimacy provides a sense of security about the relationship. It calms the individuals—provides solace. Intimacy allows people to be seen, known, accepted, understood, and treated with uniqueness. This is the stuff of friendship, good parenting, and being and staying in love. Although most friendships are not bothered by eroticization of each other, most sexual partners expect to be dear friends. Dear friendships and good lovers do some of the same things for us: They stabilize us—make us feel secure, happy, good. Mental health professionals tend to describe the inner peace, solace, or contentment in other ways. We refer to greater stability, self-cohesion, self-esteem, and improved ego function.[2] When psychological intimacies disappear from previously important relationships—no matter whether they involve spouses, lovers, friends, or a parent-child unit—various anxiety, depressive, or somatic symptoms may appear.

ARE PSYCHOLOGICAL INTIMACY AND EMPATHY SYNONYMS?

Although the above is quite basic to our human psychology, psychiatry does not discuss psychological intimacy much. Much like love, the term is primarily found in women's magazines. This is instructive. Lately there has been compelling theorizing about the essential psychological styles of girls and women.[3] Women typically require more frequent psychologically intimate experiences—with each other, with children, with lovers, with husbands—than do men. They complain more often about the lack of psychological intimacy in their relationships with men. Men are more typically patterned to more autonomous operational patterns. They have trouble understanding why women complain about their lack of communicating, why they say their marriages do not contain enough intimacy. It is now more broadly recognized by mental health professionals that psychologically healthy women organize their lives to a far greater degree around relationships—to friends, family, lovers, children, and spouses—than do healthy men. Women expect themselves to be relational, to gravitate to connection, and to personally evaluate their successes in terms of psychologically intimate relationships and responsiveness to other persons' lives. Men tend to think of themselves as successful more often in terms the creation of a unique self-sufficient wage-earning self.[4] These gross generalizations about the gender differences leave room for the scientifically verified observation that no one psychological trait is the exclusive province of either gender. Men prosper in intimate relationships as well as women do, but it is the lay publications that target female readers that endlessly return to the subject.

Psychiatry and psychology discuss empathy.[5] There is no ringing agreement about what empathy actually is, but there is more acceptance that empathy is desirable and should recur in psychotherapy. It is assumed to stimulate and enable continuing healthy psychological development.[6] Empathy has been said to heal derailed narcissistic development, to enhance the sense of self, and to enable a person to participate in a mutual relationship. Empathy involves joining the experience of another person, emotionally resonating with that person by understanding some aspect of his or her subjective world. It begins with the recognition of the self in the other. Empathy is often said to involve feeling at one with another or emotionally joining the other in creating a sense of mutuality or oneness. Occasionally, empathy is credited with creating a sense of belonging to a larger universe. Recurrent empathy in psychotherapy enables the patient and the therapist to understand the similarities and the differences in each other. Empathy is an antidote for the sense of isolation.

Sound familiar? How different is the concept of empathy from psychological intimacy? Same concept, different language package? Two different ideas? Most writers on either subject give the impression that it is readily attainable. Perhaps so, within psychotherapy. But suspicion is warranted, particularly in this era of limited, problem-oriented contact between professionals and patients. Not only do our psychotherapies often fall short of recurrent empathic experiences, the personal lives of professionals, like all people, may go by for long periods of time without the scintillating connections of intimacy (or empathy).

RELATIONSHIP BETWEEN PSYCHOLOGICAL AND SEXUAL INTIMACY

Psychological intimacy lays the groundwork for select people to become lovers. It is often the trigger to the intrapsychic rearrangement process called falling in love. Once a couple becomes lovers, the sexual behavior creates a further sense of knowing each other. But it is the ready reattainment of psychological intimacy that enables them to make love again and again over time, to shed their inhibitions during lovemaking, and to eventually discover the limits of their sexual potential with one other.

In any sexual relationship, over time it becomes increasingly difficult to behave sexually together without psychological intimacy. Lovers may quickly discover that talking, communicating, or sharing how one thinks and feels about a relevant matter increases their willingness to behave sexually. Psychological intimacy, however, requires each partner to set aside time to reestablish it when the sense of unconnection or distance is felt by either of them. This can be a formidable problem for those who do not intuitively understand these ideas, cannot provide the speaking or listening requirements, are chronically overwhelmed by other external demands, or who originally could manage only a meager intimacy. As a result the sexual potential of psychological intimacy does not get realized. It is quite common for men and women to complain that there is insufficient intimacy in their lives.

Two bypass strategies within established relationships are frequently employed to attain the benefits of intimacy without the processes of speaking and listening.

1. *Mind reading.* To some extent, people are mind readers. Many spouses, for instance, are highly skilled at deducing or guess-

ing what their partners are feeling and thinking from a glance. Mind reading, as therapists dealing with silent patients can testify, has distinct limitations: Incorrect deductions are likely; only a small fraction of another person's thoughts can be deduced; the process soon becomes boring; inscrutability provokes abandoning the aspiration for psychological and physical closeness.

2. *Sexual behavior.* Many people have more faith in the power of sexual behavior than in mind reading to re-create emotional closeness. This point of view is understandable, although far from infallible. After all, sometimes even a kiss, let alone breast or genital contact, changes a relationship and creates a nonverbal yet profound sense of knowing the other person. Busy people with dwindling time and energy during their day easily come to rely on sexual interaction to re-create closeness. It works, but not invariably. It also does not work as a long-term strategy as many people have assumed. One of its dangers is that one person may think it is working while the other is certain that it is not. Such a couple usually has little capacity to talk about their differing reactions to their sexual behavior. It continues until the illusion is shattered: One person becomes recognizably sexually dysfunctional or unmistakably angry.

Sex as a substitute for psychological intimacy probably works best during early adulthood, but as most men and women age into midlife, they need better psychological conditions to make love in a way that reliably delivers both physical and psychological satisfaction. Better psychological conditions are brought about by the establishment and reestablishment of this two-person interaction that simultaneously creates solace and pleasure.

REFERENCES

1. Simon, R.I. Natural history of therapist sexual misconduct: Identification and prevention. *Psychiatric Annals* 25:90–94, 1995.
2. Frayn, D.H. Intersubjective processes in psychotherapy. *Canadian Journal of Psychiatry* 35(5): 434–438, 1990.

3. Gilligan, C. *In a Different Voice*. Harvard University Press: Cambridge, MA, 1982.
4. Jordan, J.V. *Relational Development: Therapeutic Implications of Empathy and Shame*. Stone Center Working Paper Series, Wellseley, MA, 1989.
5. Duan, C., and Hill, C.E. The current state of empathy research. *Journal of Counseling Psychology* 43(3):261–274, 1996.
6. Jackson, S.W. The listening healer in the history of psychological healing. *American Journal of Psychiatry* 149(12):1623–1632, 1992.

3

The Paradoxes of Sexual Desire

WHAT IS SEXUAL DESIRE?

It must mean something that sexual desire is much written about but few seem to agree what it is.[1,2] Perhaps one day sexual specialists will officially create an erudite definition. Such a definition would have to encompass the ebb and flow of both subjective and behavioral phenomena: sexual fantasies; sexual dreams; initiation of self-stimulation to orgasm; initiation of sexual behavior with a partner; receptivity to the partner's initiation of sexual behavior; genital sensations; and heightened responsivity to erotic cues in the environment. In the past, when I defined sexual desire as the psychobiological energy that precedes and accompanies arousal and tends to create sexual behavior, I never took the idea too seriously. For one thing, I had little idea what psychobiological energy was. For another, I could not remember a less memorable set of words. The definition was my attempt not to surrender to the widely promoted idea that sexual desire was analogous to hunger or thirst.[3] I came to respect desire's inherent complexity from trying to assist men, women, and couples who complained of deficient, excessive, or incompatible desire. I remain impressed with three major fluctuating contributants to sexual desire: biology, psychology, and socialization. But, awareness of these three contributants is only the beginning of the story; the more sophisticated next level of appreciation begins when we see that we are largely in paradox when we come to our sexual desires. First, however, to the basics.

SEXUAL DRIVE: THE BIOLOGICAL ASPECT
OF SEXUAL DESIRE

The felt bodily energy of sexual desire, that which pushes us to sexual activity without external stimulation, what is often colloquially called *horniness*, is probably the result of activation of central neural networks. Some unknown neuroendocrine orchestration process involving hormones (testosterone, estrogen, progesterone, and neurotransmitters like dopamine, serotonin, and gammaaminobutyric acid) makes us recognize ourselves as highly interested in masturbating or having sex with a partner. Some physiological process also creates disinterest, the usual state of being beyond youth. In animals from rats to primates, this network is called the *sexual drive center*. It has been located in collections of neuronal cell bodies called *nuclei* found in the anterior-medial preoptic area of the hypothalamus; these nuclei have extensive connections to the limbic system. Anatomical destruction of these nuclei stops the sexual behaviors of animals. Pharmacological treatment with neurotransmitter agonists increases sexual behaviors; the use of antagonists block them.[4, 5] The sexual drive center has been localized to the same area in humans, where it has been found to be twice the size in adult males than in adult females. A strong suggestion of a decline of the size of these hypothalamic nuclei with advancing age exists.

The usual manifestations of sexual drive in both sexes are: genital sensations associated with minor increases in genital blood flow, erotic sensitivity to others in the environment, sexual fantasies, and planning for sexual behavior. The strength and frequency of sexual drive manifestations increase dramatically after puberty and create in many people a vague discomfort caused by not behaving sexually. Such discomfort may have a distinct periodicity in adolescence and young adulthood. A person, for example, may feel horny every three days, for three days before every period, about twice a month, or whatever the case may be. People with high sex drives seem to arrange for sexual behavior frequently and feel more calm and able to concentrate on other matters after orgasm. People with low sex drives may have spontaneous sexual feelings but they can readily ignore them without feeling irritability. After blossoming in youth and young adulthood, the manifestations of sexual drive gradually diminish until they almost entirely disappear in older age. Now that physicians commonly prescribe medications that diminish the manifestations of sexual drive, we have further realized how little is known about the physiological processes that lead a person to feel spontaneous sexual desire. Suddenly, our patients are complaining that their otherwise useful medications are making them uncharacteristically comfortable without sexual behavior.

There is something basically biological about the subjective experience of desire. Its importance stems from the organizing effect that its intensity and frequency have on our personality functioning. The fact that more adolescent boys than girls masturbate and do so at a greater frequency may at least be a reflection of a greater felt impact of spontaneous arousal during these years. Although this may reflect the presence of more neurons in the sexual drive center, more testosterone bathing the brain, or the absence of progesterone, these masturbatory tendencies are the first manifestations of the dramatic sexual tensions between the sexes that will play out for many decades.

SEXUAL MOTIVE: THE PSYCHOLOGICAL ASPECT OF SEXUAL DESIRE

The manifestations of sexual drive are contained and modified within each person. Sexual feelings are just one of many matters with which a person has to simultaneously deal. These other matters are a more important determinant of the frequency of sexual behavior than the mere presence of drive. Particularly during the middle and older decades when the frequency and intensity of sexual drive manifestations lessen, the psychological aspect of sexual desire—motive—shapes whether and how we behave sexually. Motive is recognized by a person's willingness to behave sexually. Willingness involves either initiation, receptivity, or both. Although initiation is stereotypically thought of as a male characteristic and receptivity as a female characteristic, each person, regardless of gender, has moments of direct and subtle initiation and receptivity. Motive is simply the willingness to bring one's body to a particular partner for sexual purposes.

The clinical separation of motive from drive is justified by the presence of patients who have sexual drive yet are unmotivated to engage in sexual behavior with their partners—even when it seems reasonable to them. There are three commonly recurring reasons for this paradox, the first of which is obvious.

1. That determinant of motive is how the person privately regards the partner. When the partner is appraised positively, when the reattainment of psychological intimacy is easy, and the partner remains generally cooperative in the partnership, the person's willingness to behave sexually persists. Here is the obvious: When a person is able to stay in love without a major impediment, both the sexual drive and motive act synergistically. Sexual drive is directed to the partner. "She is so wonderful and wonderful to me." The converse is even more obvious: When the partner is appraised negatively, when psychological intimacy cannot be re-created, when disappointment over the partner's failure to be helpful reigns, the person often loses his or her motive to behave sexually. A woman with vaginismus discovers her husband's infidelities, "Now, making love is the last thing I want to do!" The unwillingness to bring one's body to a partner may have little to do with sexual drive manifestations—the person may still continue to recognize sexual drive manifestations. Sexual drive and motive are in opposition.

2. The second and more subtle contributant to motive is the presence of compatibility of sexual identity. The continuation of lovemaking in a couple implies that their sexual identities are not in conflict. Many individuals lose their motive to behave sexually with their partner because they privately prefer either: (a) to personally assume a different gender, (b) to be with a partner of a different sex, or (c) to engage in an unconventional sexual behavior. Sexual identity incompatibilities efficiently generate opposition between drive and motive.

3. The third, and most subtle, contributant to motive is transference. Ideally, in a love relationship, the partner is highly valued for his or her own traits. If transferences have occurred from parents or former lovers, they are positive. For example, if a husband's devotion and loyalty reminds a wife of her parents' dedication to her, her love for him may gather momentum from her perception that he is a trustworthy nurturer just

like her parents. Clinicians are confronted with their patients' irrational attitudes toward their spouses. The patients feel anxious, untrusting, hostile, and sexually avoidant even though they positively appraise the spouse, are able to talk intimately, and generally experience the partner as cooperative. In these situations, the therapist is reminded that attitudes toward a sexual partner are composed of both real and transferential characteristics, both of which feel real. The recognition that negative transferences can create an unwillingness to behave sexually with an otherwise beloved partner removes any illusion that the motive to behave sexually is a simple matter. It is now commonly believed in our culture, for example, that forgotten, dimly remembered, or shame-ridden recall of parental sexual abuse may paralyze the person's motive to behave sexually with a loved partner. It is even assumed that either the memory of abuse per se or the emotions felt during the abuse are reexperienced during sexual behavior. Unwillingness to behave sexually with the valued partner then is explained by the fear of the remembrance.

Willingness to behave sexually reflects a positive appraisal of the partner, a sensed compatibility of sexual identity needs, and either positive transferences or the absence of negative ones. Not only does an appreciation of these factors help to explain the common problems of unwillingness to behave sexually in the population, they illuminate how sexual drive manifestations can be dwarfed by the greater power of psychological factors to determine partner sexual behavior.

SEXUAL WISH: THE SOCIAL DIMENSION OF SEXUAL DESIRE

Historians, sociologists, philosophers, theologians, and anthropologists each remind clinicians that sexual life is influenced by forces that surround the individual and are more important than the biological or psychological details of the person's life. Some early Christian sects, for example, considered sex to be a demonic evil that had to be constantly fought against through repudiation of bodily desires and sensations. The flesh was evil. The legacy of such ideas goes far beyond the few individuals who managed to live ascetically so as to overcome their desire: They have lesser manifestations in many people who live during and after the time the ideas are in ascendancy.

All sexual behaviors occur within a social field that extends from the person, to the family, to the couple, the community, the region, the nation, and time in history. These social influences mysteriously find their way to personal expectations about sexual behavior.

Sexual wishes are readily confused with motives to behave sexually because they, too, can be powerful. Wishes, however, range in power from the trivial lies we tell ourselves about our sexual lives—"I want to have sexual intercourse three times a week"—to unfortunate matters of conscience that constrain sexual behavior for a lifetime—"Nice women do not enjoy sexual life for themselves; they provide for their husbands," or "Masturbation is a sin for which you will burn eternally in Hell." These ideas are part of the socialization processes in the person's youth.

Chief among the subtle but powerful personal expectations about sex that have an enormous hold on us are those that derive from the patriarchal organization of culture. Patriarchy inconspicuously defines roles on the basis of gender rather than on the basis of a person's interests and abilities. Some couples only have intercourse in the missionary position because the man-on-top feels "normal." Some men will stimulate women but will not passively accept any sensual attention because it is not "natural." Such ideas come from the person's interpretation of the organization of culture.

A hundred years ago, educated persons considered the oral stimulation of genitals to be a form of sickness. Today, the more education people have, the more endorsing they are of personal oral genital experience. Time changes our views of what is proper sexual behavior.

Sexual wishes operate through the willingness to bring the body to sexual behavior. Unlike motive, which is more a question of "Do I participate?" sexual wishes generate different questions: "How do I participate? Do I enjoy myself? Do I devote myself solely to my partner's pleasure?" Although drive and motive may synergistically push a person to sexual behavior, some culturally acquired idea of propriety may diminish how the resulting desire is expressed.

Case Histories

Most of the vignettes presented throughout this book will consist of two parts: enough background to understand the patient's situation and dialogue between the patient and me during one session only. The cases are presented in this manner to clinically illustrate the concepts considered in the preceding paragraphs and to demonstrate how therapists might want to use the concepts in their therapeutic dialogue with patients.

Case One: A Mid-Life Moral Dilemma in a Long-Difficult Marriage

Jack is the husband of a patient I have been seeing for three years. I have seen him twice before: at the couple's initial evaluation for her chronic depression, substance abuse, and sexual aversion and about a year later when he wanted to talk to me about his continuing sexual deprivation, "even though her anxiety and depression are much better." Jack is a conspicuously kind gentle respectful man, slow to be skeptical about doctors, whose adoptive parents are both long dead. He has only one sibling—a ne'er-do-well brother who appeared again a decade ago and engaged in sex with his wife. Her symptoms increased dramatically after this in-house two-day affair. Jack quietly asked his brother to leave and said very little to my patient except, "You're sick." Jack's pleasures include his business, golf, wife, and son. He is free of psychiatric symptoms. His wife is chronically ill with depression, osteoporosis, general osteoarthritis, and medication-induced gastritis. Although she has an intense aversion to sex with her husband, based on father incest between ages 6 and 8, her lifelong private erotic "on fire" state shifted focus during our psychotherapy from the teenage boy, whose baby she gave up for adoption at age 17, to me, who understands the tragedy of her life.

Jack created a crisis when he recently told her that he wanted a separation. She panicked; much of her improvement disappeared. After one of her sullen evenings filled with angry tears, he announced that he wanted to talk it over with me and afterward he would inform her of his decision. She called and asked, "Could you see Jack soon, pleeease?"

Doctor, I don't know what to do. I told her I wanted to leave but I'm afraid that she can't manage. I see her walking up and down those stairs, she is so slow and weak. I want to move to a one level house because our house is too much for her to manage. She refuses, and says that I am crazy and that she can manage. But believe me, doctor, it is too much for her. And sex is a joke. When she feels guilty or senses that I am annoyed because it has been over a month or so, she will have sex. I'm happy to have it, I'm not really complaining...[big sigh].... except it does not happen enough.

You know I have been trying to help her with this for a long time. I wish I could tell you that she will be better and you will eventually have a reasonably normal sexual life. I think I explained this to you the last time you were here alone: Her childhood sexual experiences with her father have led her to make you into the good father. Sex with her husband causes her to be anxious like she is reliving the experience with her father. She prefers you to be good, that is, not to want to have sex with her. It is quite unfair. You did nothing wrong yet you bear the consequences of his acts.

I know she really can't get much better but I just want her to be a bit more reasonable. She is sometimes impossibly stubborn.

Well, we both have experience with that. Jack, you are such a patient man. It is both your strong suit and your weakness. You bury your resentment most of the time and recently you erupted like Mt. St. Helens.

I don't think I was serious when I said I'm going to separate. But **she** started looking for an apartment. She can be so difficult. I can't let her live alone.

So what are you doing about your sexual frustration?

I don't think about it that much. I work, and with spring coming soon I'll be on the links. That helps a lot. I don't like to masturbate too much.

Do you think about another woman?

That is just not me. I am and want to remain faithful.

When you spoke about separation, I thought maybe you just wanted to start anew with someone else.

I think about it sometimes but I could not do that to her. She is my wife. I love her, it is just that she is so impaired.

Jack, I think that you had a moral crisis. You believe in the institution of the family, you take your marital vows quite seriously, and a part of you resents the burden of her emotional impairments. She is a devoted mother and has created a family for you—something that you haven't had since you were 17 when your widowed father died. You must have been asking yourself the question, "What do I owe her?" When you think about leaving, you realize that it would be too hurtful to her for you to do, no matter how mad you feel at times. Do you see what I mean, Jack?

I can't leave her. I don't really want to. It would not be the right thing to do. What I want is to move to a more reasonable house, one that she can take care of, but she has insisted for so long on staying. It is not that important to me that we just moved into the house 18 months ago, her leg has gotten worse since then and I'm afraid she will fall down the steps.

She'll be happy to know that you have changed your mind about leaving her. Now that I think about it more, maybe your volcano erupted when you realized that it would never be much different. Maybe it was your one moment of rebellion before you settled back into your typical way of being. You made your speech and then quietly accepted your fate. You are a fine guy.

Thanks for seeing me. You know I just can't put these things into words. I know that you are right. I appreciate your help.

My pleasure Jack. Take care.

Comment: Jack manifests drive occasionally, he is generally willing to bring his body to the sexual experience with his wife whenever he feels she is not overwhelmed by the prospect. His strongest component of desire, however, is his wish to have sex. He uses this to tell himself that he is a normal man. His wife, on the other hand, has intense drives that are always maladaptively directed away from her husband. She is profoundly motivated to avoid bringing her body to him for sex and prefers to think of him as a boring lover than herself as avoiding memories of incest. She has no wish to make love to Jack. Living out these desire dynamics has generated fluctuating specific arousal and orgasmic difficulties in each person as well as significant moral paradoxes.

THE NEXT LEVEL OF SOPHISTICATION: SEXUAL DESIRE IS RIDDLED WITH PARADOX

Sexual desire introduces us to several paradoxes. Although we may announce to ourselves and our partners that we are normal and therefore have sexual desire, we generally do not like to acknowledge the high degree of conflict that the juxtaposition of drive, motive, and wish generates within us. Clinicians cannot afford the luxury of ignoring this juxtaposition paradox; it is an inherent feature of our sexuality. Most individuals deal quietly with this paradox without the language to explain what they feel and think to themselves. In the previous chapter, I emphasized that clinicians sell intimacy. Of course, this aspect of our work is only the first step that we take in creating our larger service; we provide concepts to people that help them to make sense of their mental processes. We help them to realize that their sexual desire is inherently conflictual. They may want to make love but they do not always act as though they do; they may value their sexual expression but they generally avoid it, and so forth. Drive, motive, and wish evolve in an often changing relationship to one another creating the juxtaposition paradox.

A second paradox, the fidelity paradox, arises from our affinity to marriage or prolonged couplehood. Within these committed states, men and women may periodically sexually desire someone other than their partner—even when happily situated with the partner. Although they have given up the world of other sexual partners and remain faithful, infidelity of imagination and longing continues to various degrees. Unsuppressably. Some just accept this calmly, humorously, assuming that it is just the ordinary private state of psychological being, whereas others harshly judge themselves for their failures. I think of this as the fidelity paradox. We do not give up the universe easily just for love. Besides, it may be that the hunger for idealized love that includes readily available, relaxed, sensual sexual behavior unburdened by adult responsibilities is what keeps our minds churning in this paradoxical way.

A third paradox, the lust paradox, is more private and uncomfortable. I use the term *lust* to denote the efficient, intense arousal provoked by imagery. For heterosexual men, this imagery usually is of adolescent or young adult women. Lust is stimulated by clothed or naked body parts and postures of women that suggest their desire to do the man's sexual bidding. It is important that little else about the woman be known. For a woman to provoke lust, she must be thought of as being a certain type such as attractive, eager, adventuresome, virgin; nothing much more. Lust is commonly provoked by sexual fantasy, films, reading material, and contacts with strangers. Each of these circumstances gratifies the man's seemingly insatiable curiosity about women's bodies and their private sexual behaviors. Lustful stimuli also provide a vacation from the usual complexity of actual relationships; simplicity, body parts, and the notion that the other is aching to be sexually available are all that is necessary.

Homosexual lust is the same, except that the body parts and the suggested sexual behaviors are male-centered for men and female-centered for women. Lust is usually portrayed as a male phenomenon, but women respond to imagery as well.[6] Adolescent and adult heterosexual women, for example, have body parts that are their favorites because they provide an efficient pleasure and arousal. Women are capable of longing for simple, physical sex without the usual constraints of real relationships. Women, too, can find media depictions of sexual behavior arousing. So-called female pornography, or sexually explicit imagery with a story about the women's desire, dilemmas, or relationship and less focus on penile–genital interaction, rests on the same power of body imagery to provoke excitement. Images of women who are sexually excited are sexually exciting to men and women.

Lust can be so powerful, riveting, and enjoyable that it can be experienced without paying any attention to the subtleties that allow it to emerge. But when attention is focused on the typical heterosexual variety, a power differential between the man who is being excited and the woman whose body and posturing are the source of arousal becomes apparent. Women, particularly, quickly realize the inequality in these scenes and repudiate them as degrading to women and harmful to men in allowing them to assume an unearned power in relationships devoid of attachment. The degradation and control of women in lustful images are the basis for the idea that lust contains a disguised element of aggression. Repudiated or not, containing aggression or not, it is striking how powerful such imagery can be for either sex and how these experiences may become a measuring device to use when comparing subsequent partner experiences. Some people literally become stuck at the level of pornographic depictions of sex. Pornography becomes the partnerless arena in which they play out their sexual lives.

No matter how civilized, religious, politically correct, educated, or proper we are in the conduct of our ordinary lives, the lust paradox is in us. We may desire the rich interpersonal complexities of sublime requited sensual love, but for rapid intense arousal something else can do the trick. We also routinely manage this paradox privately. Sometimes, however, the management of the lust paradox is a strong factor in threatening, limiting, or destroying relationships.

Case Two: The New Modern Desire Paradox

This is the second and final visit for this 40-year-old neatly attired trim engineer, a father of two young children. He described a steady stream of promotions at the only company he has worked for since graduation. He and his wife have a regular and mutually satisfying sexual life at least weekly. He has always been faithful without temptation. "I have a wonderful life. I am a happy person."

I was the first mental health professional seen by him. He was referred by his employee assistant program after his boss and the director of personnel confronted him about an expense irregularity. He had been using the company phone to call party lines in the Dominican Republic that hooked up people in conversation. In one month alone he made 130 separate calls. Since these calls began nine months ago, the company traced $2500 in charges. They had no complaints about his work performance and wanted this to go away very quickly. They asked for repayment, a psychiatric evaluation without their knowledge of the recommendations, a slight delay in his next expected promotion, and to be done with the issue. He was shocked at how much money and time he had spent on the phone; "This is so unlike me, I'm real careful with spending money, even the company's money." He immediately acknowledged his behavior, apologized, and quickly repaid the company. He told me that it was disturbing to realize that he had addictive behavior. This is not how he thinks of himself. Since the confrontation, he has not made another call.

He claimed that most of the actual time that he was charged for was spent waiting to be hooked up with someone. He did not notice it because he was doing his usual computer work while waiting. Approximately ten times, however, he managed to get exactly what he wanted: He spoke seductively to a real woman about his age—one who called in as he did. "I tell her a bit about myself—a lot of acting, lying is involved. I quickly let her know that she is wanted, that I intensely desire her. I try to get the woman to masturbate while talking to her and to have multiple orgasms. *I* don't masturbate."

Never in any kind of trouble, this quiet man who shares the household and childrearing chores 50:50, has no evidence of paraphilia, sexual compulsivity or dysfunction. He has never been given to any excesses, alcohol, substances of abuse, or gambling. He dated several women before his wife. Neither he nor his wife wanted children very strongly in the early marriage but now that they are here they are the joyful center of his life. He regrets working only in that it keeps him from spending more time with his kids. He thinks of himself as a relatively shy person. "I was never any good at smooth-talking any woman." Now that he is older, he is more experienced in the world and more confident. He discovered the chatting rooms on the Internet several years ago, but was not too interested. He thought much of the sex talk was crazy or from disturbed people. He was untrusting of the typed word as anyone could be pretending to be anyone else there. Last year while out of town on business, on a lark, he dialed a number he saw advertised in a magazine and found it fun and safe. It just grew from there. He sensed no alienation from his wife, no special life event that preceded the escalation, but "I had not actually realized how it had escalated—130 times in 20 workdays. Wow! It is really frightening." He had not yet told his wife about the company's confrontation. He was fearful of her responses.

How was our session two weeks ago for you?

It was helpful talking this over with you. It particularly was good that you encouraged me to tell my wife about it. It was not easy. She was shaken—but I told her everything—how it got started, what I was trying to do, what actually sometimes happened. After a few days, thankfully, she seemed more concerned about the effect on my career. I promised I would never do anything like this again. She knows that I love her.

What about the temptation to call since I saw you last?

None. I think it was like a shock therapy: it was a traumatic experience for me and for my wife. It has shaken the desire for it out of me.

So, now that it is over, what was it about really?

This must have been my form of a mid-life crisis. Strange, I'm so happy with my life, but I have to tell you that I was very impressed how I could talk to these women. No vulgarity. I could find the words. I was eloquent. I sometimes would laugh at how powerful my words were. I realized that I am much more confident now. I just could not stop seeking the pleasure of the experience. It just got the best of me. I was doing it automatically.

I remember that you said that you were a shy young man and never could sweet-talk a girl.

Well, on the party line I guess I felt I grew up and finally could do it.

Do you consider this a mild form of infidelity?

I didn't, but Betsy sure did. I told her that I am not even tempted to be unfaithful, but she was briefly real bummed out about it.

You have intimate talk with an unknown woman, tell her about how you are caressing her breasts and genitals, assist her in her imagination to have (or pretend to have) an orgasm or two, and then try to tell Betsy that you don't consider this infidelity. The mind must have some impressive power to define meanings of words.

After a few days, Betsy acknowledged that it was not the same as having an affair and she was glad that I only did that and was not actually with a woman. But, I know it was wrong because I was so frightened to tell her and hurt her.

Well, lots of people struggle to be faithful. I imagine that you, too, in your own way were struggling with the idea of an affair. You see you found a way to have an affair while not having an affair. You were technically faithful and yet you had some of the pleasures of an affair without the usual messy complications.

But I don't mind being faithful!

Paradox, eh? You act in a modern technologic version of a little dalliance, deny to yourself you are being unfaithful, keep the activity from your wife, and lose control over your usual vigilant restraint mechanisms. You, Mr. Moderation, were so attracted to the opportunity to reaffirm your now matured seductive lingo that you lost control of yourself.

I don't want to do this again. Ever!

What else is there to this problem?

There is a story that I like to tell from my childhood that I think has a bearing on this. I think that this event shaped my life. On the first day of first grade, a boy who repeated the year—a bully—invited me to sit in a chair. When I sat down, he pulled the chair from under me. Since that time trust has been very important in my life. I'm always wondering if people are trustworthy? I made that bully into my friend eventually. Somehow this is related.

How?

I'm not sure, but it was really important that those women trusted me, believed me that I wanted them. I was playing with the trust factor; could I get them to trust me with their excitement, to tell me about their fantasies, and to imagine having sex with me.

But you were lying to these women. You were like the bully, making a joke at their expense and feeling powerful as a result. You almost laughed out loud with delight about what a good talker—seducer—you were. You enjoyed the power so much.

It was not very nice when you think about it.

It was self-indulgent—simply for your pleasure.

The women were there for pleasure too. You would be surprised at how many women call into these lines for the excitement of it.

It is a growth industry. But more to the point, this pleasure envelops you in a mighty paradox. You want honesty and trust and you behave dishonestly and exploit trust for the sport of it. There is another irony here: now that you are finally able to smooth-talk, you are a well-married young middle-aged man who has no legitimate basis for using your skill. The good news is that you can finally feel good about meeting a young man's standard of masculine adequacy—you can seduce women. The bad news is that it is too late to seduce women. You're married and believe in the institution and its potentials.

Do you mean that I have to grow up and just let this go? [A funny laugh occurs indicating that he knows the answer to his question.]

Yep.

I think I already have. I like to think of myself as a good person. I don't like the embarrassment.

I think you are a fine person. You just temporarily lost your way.

It really is frightening how crazy my behavior got—130 calls in one month!

Well, go and be sane. Good luck. Come back any time you'd like.

PSYCHOLOGICAL INTIMACY, DESIRE, AND LOVE

When these three powerful notions—psychological intimacy, desire, and love—are placed side by side, mental health professionals understandably reject simplistic notions of their interrelationships. Love and psychological intimacy are ideals that, although sometimes attained to a high degree, usually are not. Sexual desire, particularly biological drives, are routine ingredients of subjective life, but their expression with a partner is often so complicated that journalists independently reinvent the cute question, "Is there sex after marriage?" Paradox-ridden sexual desire more accurately reflects the range of our human natures. Love and intimacy better illuminate the highest aspirations of our beings. But a more complete understanding of our sexual lives requires both the high and the low ends of human experience to be known and accepted. These three topics need to be considered together to better understand the struggles that human beings routinely wage within themselves.

REFERENCES

1. Kaplan, H.S. *The Sexual Desire Disorders:Dysfunctional Regulation of Sexual Motivation.* Brunner/Mazel: New York, 1995.
2. Rosen, R.C., and Lieblum, S.R. *Sexual Desire Disorders.* Guilford: New York, 1995.
3. Kaplan, H.S. *Desire Disorders:Sexual Desire: Other New Concepts and Techniques in Sex Therapy.* Brunner/Mazel: New York, 1995.
4. Pomerantz, S.M. Neurotransmitter influences on male sexual behavior of rhesus monkeys. Paper presented at IASR, August 1991, Barrie, Ontario.
5. Foreman, M.M., Hall, J.L., and Love, R.L. The role of 5-HT-2 receptor in the regulation of sexual performance of male rats. *Life Sciences* 45:1263–1270, 1989.
6. Laan, E., and Everaerd, W. Habituation of female arousal to slides and film. *Archives of Sexual Behavior* 24(5):517–541, 1995.

4

Psychological Development
in Mid-Life

> Perhaps the greatest problem faced by the
> academic social sciences is that what is
> measurable is often irrelevant and what is truly
> relevant often cannot be measured....
> —George Vaillant

INTRODUCTION

If we are to have a reasonable chance to be of assistance to individuals
passing through their fifth and sixth decades of life, we have to be pre-
pared to think and speak from three platforms of knowledge: biology,
individual psychological development, and relationship evolution.
Each of these topics is formulated by different disciplines. The biology
of physically healthy mid-life is primarily of concern to physicians
who deal with menopausal complaints. Individual adult maturation is a
subject most commonly invoked by psychoanalysts. It has been more
scientifically detailed, however, by prospective cross-sectional studies
of adults that have been conducted by researchers interested in building
conceptual models of development. Comparatively little work has been
done on the subject of relationship evolution despite the fact that many
clinicians deal with relationship problems.

GENERAL ISSUES

Definitions of Psychological Development and Maturation

Psychological development or maturation is a natural personal change process that leads to new forms of behavior and new functions. Changes occur in emotional reactivity, thinking, interests, meanings given to events, values, ambitions, life style, taste (aesthetics), spirituality, the use of defense mechanisms, and self-concepts.

Maturational changes seem to occur as a result of interactions of three inexorable forces: biology, mental activity, and environmental demands. The ultimate mechanisms that bring them about are unseen and perhaps unknowable.

Do Healthy Adults Continually Develop?

Some disagreement exists about the answer to this question. The disagreement stems from differing notions about the causes of adult emotional difficulties.

The "No" Position

Four decades ago, most mental health professionals were taught that psychological development ended with adolescence. The term *adult development* made little conceptual sense and was not commonly used. Adulthood was thought to consist of a long stable period during which dramas of marriage and career unfolded and a shorter degenerative period during which aging and disease dominated intrapsychic and interpersonal life. Childhood conflicts were enduring, although often unconsciously rearranged, and expressed through adult disguises. These childhood-derived conflicts were thought to be lingering vulnerabilities to adult decompensations that could readily reemerge to generate mental suffering throughout adulthood. Many therapists felt that psychodynamic therapy was the only way to reverse the damage of early life development. Some thought that damage was inevitable.

The "Yes" Position

Different assumptions are operative today. This may be because of an increased cultural sophistication about the multiple determinants of mental life, the waning influence of psychoanalytic ideas on the education of mental health professionals, or intellectual fashion. Mental health professionals now tend to believe that psychological development continues throughout adulthood. Individuals have the potential to grow psychologically to evolve new mental capacities in response to the demands of their adult roles. People do not develop smoothly, linearly, continuously. They mature asynchronously. Adult experiences can generate symptoms regardless of childhood experience. Given enough time and life experience, even the immature often change in basic ways, particularly if the impediments to their maturation such as substance abuse, depression, or loneliness can be removed. There are many avenues to maturation besides therapy. Therapy is not even the most common catalyst of psychological development.

Is Development Relevant to Mental Health Professionals?

The "Yes, of Course!" Position

Mental health professionals routinely perform four roles: diagnostician, compassionate companion of the mentally distressed, agent of symptom relief, and behavioral change catalyst. An understanding of adult development is background preparation for each of these roles because notions about how individuals develop, or fail to develop, may be ultimate explanations for the pathogenesis of symptoms. This statement is so rudimentary to some professionals that it seems insulting to belabor: "Of course, failed development is the cause of psychopathology!" These professionals tend to assume that developmental conflict is almost everything in terms of understanding mental life. They also tend to assume that adequate therapy causes maturation.

The "Maybe" Position

The idea that the study of development is relevant for something other than preparatory education is revolutionary to some in our field. It is, at best, only a hypothesis waiting to be tested. These professionals emphasize the differences between distress and disorder, between difficulties in living and psychopathology. They rely on data-bound science as the final arbiter of fact. They may not be able to address topics that are currently larger than the scientific method can encompass. For them, theories about development are just unverifiable uncertainties that harken back to the era of descriptive prescientific psychiatry. To the extent that developmental issues are only cofactors in the production of a particular psychopathology, this camp may be simultaneously right and wrong.

Newer Ideas among Psychoanalysts

Some psychoanalysts have been recently stressing that adults develop.[1] Their notions challenge the assumption that almost everything vital to psychodynamic life is set up early in development. Here are some of the newer ideas:

- Development is essentially the same in childhood and adulthood—both are deeply dependent on their environment. In all phases of life, individuals must engage in and master developmental tasks such as sexual function, intimacy, creativity, work, and loss.
- Development is an ongoing dynamic process in which new capacities evolve from those that first appeared in childhood and adolescence.
- Childhood issues, which remain a central aspect of adult psychological life, do not entirely explain adult life. Experiences during young or middle years are also potent influences on the adult.
- Biological decline, culminating in the awareness of the finiteness of time and the inevitability of death, is an important part of almost all of adult life.

Each of these concepts pays homage to psychoanalytic theory, which teaches that children are preoccupied with definable intrapsychic tensions while traversing their developmental stages. Child development stresses what children have in common rather than the differences among them as they enter, deal with, and resolve their predictable preoedipal, oedipal, latency, and adolescent issues.

Adult Development Is Different

Development of the adult has long been recognized as different from that of childhood. As far as we can tell, infants are more alike than different. By the time 21 years has passed, differences among young adults are quite evident. By the time adults are middle-aged, their differences are further magnified. Development is a process of progressive differentiation or, as mental health professionals are used to writing, individuation. Differentiation has three times longer to occur during adulthood. The young (20–39), middle (40–59), later (60–79), and late-late adulthood (80+) eras are almost each as long as childhood and adolescence. It is an easier task to describe the substages of 20 years than of 60 years. Schoolchildren are grouped by age and can be more easily studied. Their predictable physical development generates natural stages of psychological development. Little interest exists in the physical changes that normally occur as healthy adults age.

ERIKSON'S MONUMENTAL CONCEPTS OF DEVELOPMENT

Table 1 presents Erikson's now-classic sequences of childhood and adult development[2] and has been modified according to Vaillant's division of young adulthood into two eras.[3] The last column contains the trait that is thought to emerge from mastery of the developmental de-

Table 1. Erikson's Model of the Life Cycle

Approximate age	Psychoanalytic labels	Developmental challenges	Acquired ideal trait
First year of life	Oral stage	Basic trust vs. mistrust	Hope
Years 2 and 3	Anal stage	Autonomy vs. shame	Will
Years 3 to 6	Oedipal stage	Initiative vs. guilt	Purpose
Years 7 to puberty	Latency stage	Industry vs. inferiority	Competence
Adolescence	Adolescence	Identity vs. identity diffusion	Fidelity
Years 21 to 30	Young adulthood	Intimacy vs. isolation	Love
Years 30 to 40	Young adulthood	Career consolidation vs. self-absorption	Competence, commitment, contentment, compensation
Years 40 to 60	Middle age	Generativity vs. stagnation	Care
Years 60–80	Older age	Integrity vs. despair	Wisdom

mands of each phase. The consequences of not adequately meeting these challenges can be found following the "vs." in the third column.

When Erikson described the large developmental challenges for each stage of life—for instance, mid-life stagnation versus generativity—he considered the conflicts and developmental issues in young, middle, and older ages to be universal, genetically grounded, sequential, yet heavily interactive with the environment. He termed the evolution of developmental conflict and opportunity *epigenesis*. He warned that if the age-expectant conflicts are not optimally resolved during the correct epigenetic era, further development is jeopardized.

Students of adult development now think that individual lives are marked by different spheres of psychological function. These spheres advance, stagnate, or regress at separate rates. In this way, child and adult development are similar, but adults have more functions, more roles, more opportunities for success and failure than children. When we speak of middle age, it is possible to sketch in Eriksonian fashion a series of general issues that typically are being dealt with by people between ages 40 and 60. But although most 40-year-olds may be dealing with a particular issue—parenting for instance—the specifics of their challenges vary considerably. At age 40, some women have raised their children while others are having their first baby. Their 15-year-olds may be boys, girls, retarded, gifted, twins, adopted, or one of many children. When theorizing, we may speak of parenting teenagers as a developmental challenge but the difference in the specific challenges can easily be overlooked.

DEVELOPMENTAL TASKS

Definition

This term refers to any psychological challenge that demands accommodation. The challenge may be conceived of either as universal, such as learning how to manage money, or as unique to the person, such as learning how to manage life on very little money. If the person deals with the challenge well, our field has agreed to say the person *masters* the task. As a direct consequence of mastery, self-confidence is enhanced, the person acquires new information, awareness, and behavior, and is afforded new life opportunities—the person matures. Here is a common example of mastering a specific parental developmental middle-age task. A 40-year-old man leaves his wife and daughter. This weighty decision and its aftermath have left him in turmoil. His daughter is not eager to be with him, and he would just as soon avoid her adolescent moodiness and embarrassment about being seen with him. Nonetheless, his parental obligation and aspiration to not abandon his child enable him to deal with the long period of unpleasantness. Eventually, being with her is easy and often enjoyable. She and he come to value their connection and now vacation together eagerly. Years later, each feels that the other was an important ingredient in getting through the adverse times. During her college years, they privately feel that they love each other in the best sense of father–daughter love.

A developmental task is designated as such because it is something that does not go away. If the person deals with it poorly or avoids dealing with it, the issue remains to shape feelings and thoughts and to limit behaviors and possibilities. If a man, for instance, is too ashamed of having left his family to see his child regularly, too often incensed that his wife has poisoned his daughter against him, too angry at his daughter's insensitivity to his pain, the developmental demand to parent remains whether he sees his daughter or not. Whichever way the forces in this dissolving family align, he, his daughter, and his ex-wife will be shaped by his ability to master the demands for parenting from outside the daughter's home.

Limitations of the Concept of Developmental Tasks

1. *General versus specific tasks.* If we define developmental tasks as universal themes that engage almost every adult at a particular time of life, we, of necessity, speak in generalities. If we define developmental tasks by looking at the specific challenges of an individual's life, we speak through case histories or biographies. Each has its rewards and limitations. During the middle years, most people have to deal with: the physiological declines of early aging; increased awareness of time limitation and personal death; illness and death of par-

ents, friends, and relatives; changes in sexual drive and activity; changes in relationships to parents, children, and spouse; assessment of career accomplishments, planning for retirement. If we eavesdrop on the conversations of the middle-aged, these are the subjects that we will often hear them discussing. The middle-aged are simultaneously dealing with many separate developmental tasks; each task undergoes significant change over the 20 years between age 40 and 60.

2. *The relative nature of success.* Clinicians should not take the idea of mastery or failure of a task too seriously. Mastery is a linguistic creation of our psychological professions—it is only jargon. In reality, there are many forms of developmental successes each with a subtly different, good-enough outcome. There are many forms of failure as well, each with subtly different, less-than-adequate outcome that limit the person's future. The variety of outcomes of any particular developmental task assists us in appreciating how individual personhood is.

3. *Events do not often happen in an ideal sequence.* Neither should the time sequence of what challenges people be taken too literally. Erikson's model assumes many forces are being held constant. What happens when is shaped by variables belonging to the individual such as biological health, the environment the person helped to shape because of personal psychological style, as well as forces beyond the individual—family, job market, and war, to name a few. A parent becomes disabled, for instance, and needs an adult child to be the caretaker. This may occur during young, middle, older age, or never. Having to be a caregiver at age 21 is vastly different than at age 61. Individual differences in the perception of a task to be mastered must also be considered. Whether the adult child will respond to this parental need at all should not be assumed.

4. *People play catch-up.* Commonly, individuals in any particular decade are still working on accomplishing the tasks from the previous one. Our theories do not include an understanding of the effects of unmastered tasks on the already accomplished ones. As a result, the outcome of development can be quite surprising.

5. *Not all developmental failures create the same impact.* Certain failures are more destructive than others. Some common

events such as divorce or serious physical illness consume so much energy, attention, and consideration that other possibilities for adult development are routinely delayed. Other events are merely temporarily stressful. Even in the case of similar life problems, however, differences in psychological outcome are great.

6. *Men have received more attention in these studies.* Developmental tasks and their sequences tend to be presented as though they apply equally to both men and women, but there is a possibility that male bias has crept into their formulation. For instance, generativity—nurturing co-workers, giving to the community, helping the young, generally caring for others—is not something that women finally learn during their middle years!

7. *All models are limited.* Here are three great questions:

- Who does well in life?
- Who does not?
- What explains the differences?

The developmental task model is only one of several seeking to account for our fate as individuals. Model builders are quick to point out that all models are limited in their abilities to definitively answer these questions, in part because of methodological flaws, in part because the questions are too large, in part because there are too many aspects to any one human being. The models that mental health professionals may briefly encounter during their education include: Erikson's life cycle, Piaget's cognitive development, Loevinger's ego development, and Kohlberg's moral development. Each exists because it explains some aspects of psychological maturation. But although they are each scientifically supported and correspond somewhat to each other, they are only models.

Developmental Tasks by Decade

Adolescence

Here is a rephrasing of Hamburg's summary of 10 tasks that adolescents must accomplish to be healthy[4]:

1. Find a valued place in a constructive group

   2. Learn how to form durable, close relationships

   3. Feel a sense of self-worth

   4. Attain a reliable basis for making choices

   5. Learn how to use the various support systems that are available to them

   6. Display constructive curiosity and exploratory behavior

   7. Believe in a promising future with real opportunities

   8. Learn how to be useful to others

   9. Learn how to live respectfully with others in a democratic pluralism

  10. Cultivate the inquiring and problem-solving skills that serve lifelong learning and adaptability

Twenties

During the 20s, individuals expand their base of competent independence while searching for sex, intimacy, love, commitment, and vocational opportunity. During this decade, successful people move from their potentiality to early realization.

   1. Completion of adolescent tasks

   2. Increasing emotional independent self-regulation

   3. Clarification of vocational aspirations and skill development

   4. Identification of an acceptable partner

   5. Learning how to be lovingly interactive and committed to the partner

   6. Increasing financial independence

Thirties

During the 30s, besides playing catch-up for undone tasks of the 20s, many people are refining their skills in the various roles begun in their 20s—being a spouse or partner, working, parenting, creating a social network, coming to grips with the realities of one's financial present and likely future, juggling too much most of the time. The 30s are about ambition, refining success, and fatigue.

   1. Refinement of parenting capacities

   2. Refinement of vocational skills

   3. Refinement of financial independence

    4. Refinement of capacity to be intimate physically and psycho-
logically
    5. Balancing obligations to friends, career, family, and extended
family
    6. Preserving physical health

Forties

During this decade, many people are starting over—in a career, in
a marriage, with stepchildren, or in sobriety. The previous experiences
of raising children notwithstanding, parents are bracing themselves for
the challenges of their adolescents. People who have been successful at
work are making the transition to managerial roles, setting policy, and
learning about the higher levels of functioning where they work. Concerns for money are high, as are expenditures. Life has long ago become serious; personal and spousal limitations are generally evident. A
deeper grasp of life seems to be emerging. The form and function of the
body, which may have been things of beauty, are waning. The body's
vulnerability to illness, accident, and poor health habits is now harder
to ignore.

    1. Preparing for greater independence from children
    2. Assuming power in the workplace
    3. Starting a second career for mothers who stayed home to raise
children
    4. Taking stock, planning, and doing something about financial
situation
    5. Planning for the remaining years of life
    6. Remaking of self-concept in terms of early aging
    7. Taking care of the physical self
    8. Dealing with declining parents

Fifties

During the 50s, the period of graying, balding, and enlarging girth,
successful people exercise more power at work. Children emancipate
themselves or fail to do so. Money and retirement planning are being
discussed. Death has usually visited acquaintances, relatives, and an occasional friend, making one more earnest about health maintenance.

Women deal with gynecological changes and hot flashes while men notice their diminishing sex drives. Parents, even the healthy ones, are becoming frail, which leads to an ever-greater personal preoccupation with health and maintaining vitality.

1. Preserving health so that one can continue on
2. Nurturing others at the workplace
3. Consolidating financial resources for the retirement years
4. Exercising power at work
5. Pursuing nonvocational pleasures
6. Finding new interests, ambitions, activities, friends
7. Dealing with adult children
8. Exploration of psychological and sexual intimacy at a slower, less intense pace

DEVELOPMENTAL LINES

The lists of developmental tasks provide an introduction to the constantly evolving contexts of adult lives. Often the changes are slow; sometimes they are precipitous. The lists describe the arenas in which most people are challenged to develop competencies: independence, couplehood, parenting, vocational evolution, financial management, health maintenance, friends, community, recreation, and parents.

On the surface, at least, a developmental task might be relatively quickly mastered. A young person gets a job that pays enough money to support a modest life and manages to live within the limits of the paycheck. The middle-aged parents are now free of the financial need to support. The young person's self-concept is enhanced. What went into developing the ability to work and manage money and what the person is going to do with the demands of the job tomorrow are not apparent from knowing that the task was mastered. The concept of the developmental line enables an appreciation of the answers to such questions.

Definition

Each of the arenas of life in which a person develops over a long period of time is a developmental line. Sexuality, financial management, and vocational evolution, for instance, may each be considered a developmental line. The use of developmental lines implies a long-term perspective about related tasks over several decades. The use of the concept helps to clarify how one accomplishment positions a person for another.

Thinking about developmental lines affords clinicians opportunities to get beyond the *history of the present illness* to a relevant *past history* and to thinking about the patient's future. The clinician chooses a developmental line and asks intelligent questions that highlight what went before the present situation. As this is done, the hypothesis that the patient's symptoms bear some relationship to developmental considerations can be weighed.

This approach matures the clinician. It forces professionals to see that people are simultaneously successes and failures and have elements of immaturity along side solidly mature functioning. It assists us to clearer, more realistic thinking—our never completely mastered professional developmental challenge. Clinicians have a tendency to overemphasize the importance of useful psychiatric ideas and to consider them verifiably correct. Working with these large ideas about adult development exposes us to their limitations. It can help us more humbly understand the important but limited goals of much of psychotherapy:

- To help master some developmental task
- To facilitate progress along one developmental line
- To alleviate some symptomatic emotional state so that the natural process of development can proceed

These three tasks do not resemble the therapeutic goals of many of our psychiatric forebears who thought they were remaking their patients' personalities.

Imagine a Figure

To conceptualize the complexity of any person's life in developmental terms, one need only imagine each developmental line pictured side by side in a bar graph arrangement. For every person the height of each of the bars will be somewhat different. But what cannot be graphically illustrated is the influence of each of the developmental lines on the other. One might be able to say that a young woman who has mastered each of her tasks reaches an ideal state where almost everything that she does facilitates everything else. Similarly, one might say that failure breeds more failure. But within these two unusual extremes, it remains uncertain how one success or failure influences the person's approach to the future. It is possible that developmental lines reverberate to facilitate or inhibit future accomplishments. I don't know how to illustrate this in a figure.

Vaillant on Erikson's Model

Vaillant has used empirical data from three longitudinal studies to support Erikson's model. In *The Wisdom of the Ego,* he summarized data from both sexes, in two social classes, and found that the original descriptions of the major issues at stake were well captured by Erikson. This included the consequences of successes and failures. He, too, affirmed that the tasks have to be mastered in order for the person to accomplish increasingly complex integration.

Vallaint modified the Erikson model because he perceived that the 30s were a vital time for career consolidation. By career he meant having a vocational identity that both the individual and society value. The hallmarks of career consolidation were competence, commitment, contentment, and compensation. These can be seen in motherhood and homemaking and in the external workplace. Men have an easier time of it, however. Whereas they can readily follow the pathway from apprenticeship to craftsman between 20 and 40 years of age, women's career pathways are often far more arduous, less orderly, and restricted.

Vaillant uses the phrase *keeper of the meaning* to capture Erikson's mid-life generativity. Generativity is characterized by an appreciation of irony and ambiguity, justice, and caring about the world's people and environments. A keeper of meaning is concerned with giving to others—mentoring, community involvement—and to the culture.

Looking at development longitudinally and with people who are not necessarily patients, he offers three explanations for how the usually smooth transitions of development become symptomatic crises.

- Psychopathology—something within people early in life that continues to limit them during adulthood. For instance, troubled adolescents are also likely to be troubled 40-year-olds.

- The failure to adequately ritualize key transitions such as marriage, retirement, death.
- The occurrence of life transitions out of expected sequence. For example, widowhood is a greater crisis at age 40 than at age 80 (This is an obscure way of saying bad luck.)

Maturation and the Mechanisms of Defense

Vaillant has long been interested in the mechanisms of defense.[5] His most recent discussion of this basic traditional topic again is cogent, sophisticated, research-supported, and increases our understanding of how coping, creativity, adaptation, and maturation occur. Despite the compelling nature of his observations, the mystery of the maturational process remains.

He stresses that his notions represent one of many versions of the defenses. Defenses, partially seen by their users, distort both inner and outer reality. Depending on the preponderance of their use, defenses either help or hinder our adaptation to life. Those who use higher level defenses have a far greater likelihood of less troubled adult lives. Here are his categories:

- Five *mature defenses*—altruism, sublimation, suppression, anticipation, and humor
- Four *neurotic defenses*—displacement, isolation/intellectualization, repression, and reaction formation
- Six *immature defenses*—projection, fantasy, hypochondriasis, passive-aggression, acting out, and dissociation
- Three *psychotic defenses*—delusional projection, denial, and distortion

Healthier defenses enable mastery of new intrapsychic or external situations by:

1. Reducing the intensity of feelings
2. Channeling the expression of feelings elsewhere
3. Improving the chances for dealing with the future
4. Being specific to the problem being coped with
5. Attracting rather than repelling others

Over time, the preponderant use of defenses should evolve toward the more mature ones. As people grow older, they are supposed to recognize their problems as internal rather than external and to stop feeling guilty about instinctual conflicts.

Vaillant's data strongly suggest that maturity, virtue, and mental health are inextricably related. The use of defenses can also be witnessed in creative, talented, intellectually gifted people as well as more ordinarily endowed humans. In all of us, the defenses are how we mold the conditions of our lives to make them more bearable. Clinical studies of any particular person yield an appreciation of the predominant use of a defense or two. But what drives these transitions in our lives? What is the engine for development? Choices for the answers to this question overlap, compete, and are basically only models:

- The inexorability of genetic programming of the growth and unfolding of the central nervous system's capacities
- The programming effect of family life experience on the behavioral patterns and capacities of children and adolescents
- The inherent capacities of the person to be changed by life experience—particularly the experience of loving other people

As Vaillant explores the various processes of connecting with and taking in other people, there is no doubt where he stands on the question of whether adults develop. Undoubtably we do, if we are lucky, talented, or expose ourselves to the lives of others and the institutions of culture.

WHAT SHOULD BE IN PLACE BY MID-LIFE?

Here is a safe answer to this question: Maturity, the term that always recurs in discussions of development, ideally should be evident by midlife. What is it? There are innumerable ways of answering this question. Peck[6] offered four accomplishments that indicate "maturity":

- Valuing wisdom over physical strength and attractiveness
- Socialization as a replacement for sexualization of relationships
- Flexibility in shifting to new people, activities, and roles
- Mental flexibility in approaching new situations

Vaillant had much to say:

- Having appropriate expectations and goals for oneself
- Finding a major source of fulfillment in work
- The capacity to love and to hope
- The ability to discharge hostility without harming others or oneself
- The capacity to suspend one's adult identity and engage in childlike play
- The capacity to sustain paradox because the person now senses life's inherent ambiguity, knows that he or she possesses and must reconcile inner conflict, understands that love and friendship demand the ablty to cherish another's individuality even when one does not entirely agree with it
- A defensive alignment that maintains a creative and flexible tension between irreconcilables. The mature person at mid-life allows conscience, impulse, reality, and attachment to coexist at center stage.

Jung thought that maturity consisted of the integration of conflicting tendencies of the personality.[7] Middle age was the time people could be mature, that is, turn from social interests and activities to inner, spiritual, religious, philosophical issues. Middle-aged people could finally integrate unconscious experience into everyday life and begin to develop patience and wisdom. Such maturity was the beginning of the ability to identify with all living things in an uncritical appreciative way.

Stevens-Long provided several dimensions of maturity at this phase of life[8]:

- *In terms of motivation*, self-actualized generativity is characterized by the need to develop and maintain a social system; to continue to individuate; to be stable and responsible in the face of pressure.
- *In terms of emotion*, the ability to maintain a sense of self and to exercise good judgment, compassion, and control despite personal and social disequilibrium.
- *In terms of cognition*, the ability to compare relationships across systems, and to find adequate solutions.

- *In terms of behavior,* to be productive without wasted effort, all
  the while evidencing compassion for others.

Maslow's concept was that in mid-life, a mature person is self-actualized, problem-centered as opposed to self-centered, committed to the benefit of others, and capable of intense, profound relationships.[9] Only when more basic needs have been met—safety, belonging, love, and self-esteem—could the person finally fulfill his or her creative potential. Such a self-actualized person is discriminating and can now better see the truth, detect fakery and dishonesty, and can accept the self, others, and nature.

Can these varied concepts of mid-life maturity be summarized? Should we at least expect the mature to have insight into themselves and others, be capable of logical problem solving, be able to love other people, to have interests beyond themselves, and sense something grander in operation in the universe than their personal concerns? The developmental issues involved with conceptualizing mid-life have been most comprehensively presented in a book by Stevens-Long and Commons.[10]

Love and Development

Models and experts aside, science, clinical experience, parenting, and common sense converge to generate the idea that development is a complex interaction of biology, environment, individual psychology, and luck. Even if the autonomous generator of development is merely genetically driven, it seems clear to this author that some factors from each of these four categories facilitate the smooth developmental progressions and others interfere with human potentiality mightily.

Whether we are discussing intimacy in the Eriksonian manner or as in Chapter 2, whether we acknowledge the powerful potential role of sexual behavior to create and cement attachment bonds or leave it out of our models for development, the discussion is heading in the same direction. *There are ways to be with people that promote attachment, that periodically stimulate emotions that are interpreted as love, that generate respect for the person's individuality, and that lead to a self-soothing and growth-promoting internalization of the other—ways that promote our developmental potential.*[11] Sadly, it is the absence of such psychosocial environments, impairments in biological capacities, and bad luck that are the leading explanatory candidates for mental suffering and failure to develop personal potential on time. To complicate the issue further, some of these negative conditions also have the capacity to stimulate maturity. And this, coping well with adversity, at all stages of life is the greatest developmental challenge.

By mid-life, it is hoped that individuals have figured out how to be kind, supportive, and nurturing so that they can have an easier time in the remainder of their lives. If they have not and they encounter a mental health professional, one of us is likely to perceive the presence of psychopathology.

Simple and Complicated Paradoxes

Developmental theorists speak of the middle of life as the time when the person learns to contain, balance, or integrate the contradictory aspects of his or her behavior. These contradictions are sometimes seen as:

- Ambivalences of emotion such as loving and feeling deeply disappointed about a parent's character
- Conflicting loyalties to dual ambitions such as to family and work
- Genuine-appearing/ungenuine feeling such as caring for a friend as long as the social rewards persist

Such paradoxes are the relatively easy ones. Their management is an everyday part of life at every adult stage. At mid-life, more people see that their contradictions exist and have learned to manage them more calmly with the tools that they have acquired over time.

Paradox has other unattractive, far more complicated forms that often culminate in mid-life dramas. Deceit, manipulation, infidelity, lying, thievery, fraud, unethical behavior also pose developmental challenges. Perhaps these come from past developmental failures, I am not certain. Some people easily contain their dishonesties, others suffer from their conscience, and some others do a little of both. The dishonesties that mental health professionals are called on frequently to deal with involve sex, love, intimacy, and marriage. Complicated paradoxes do not often appear in our models of adult development. They routinely appear in our practices.

When we were younger mental health professionals, we tended to not perceive the paradoxes very quickly because we thought we were to make a diagnosis and provide one of the modern treatments of our day. But professionals become middle-aged too and with maturation comes a basic questioning. Our professional developmental line probably goes from enthusiastic faith in our newly learned concepts, to gradual doubting of these given-from-on-high notions, to a balanced assessment of strengths and weaknesses. Hopefully cynicism does not totally overtake the process.

REFERENCES

1. Nemiroff, R.A., and Colarusso, C.A. (eds.). *New Dimensions in Adult Development.* Basic Books: New York, 1990, pp. 97–124.
2. Erikson, E.H. *Childhood and Society*, 2nd ed. Norton: New York, 1963
3. Vaillant, G.E. *The Wisdom of the Ego.* Harvard University Press: Cambridge, MA, 1993.
4. Hamburg, D.A. Towards a strategy for healthy adolescent development. *American Journal of Psychiatry* 154(6)Festschrift Supplement:7–12, 1997.
5. Vaillant, G.E., Bond, M., and Vaillant, C.O. An empirically validated hierarchy of defense mechanisms. *Archives of General Psychiatry* 43:786–794, 1986.
6. Peck, R. Psychological development in the second half of life. In: B.L. Neugarten (ed.), *Middle Age and Aging.* University of Chicago Press: Chicago, 1968, pp. 88–96.
7. Jung, C.G. *Modern Man in Search of a Soul.* Harcourt, Brace & World: New York, 1933.
8. Stevens-Long, J. Adult development: Theories past and future. In: R.A. Nemiroff and C.A. Colarusso (eds.), *New Dimensions in Adult Development.* Basic Books: New York, 1990, pp. 125–165.
9. Maslow, A.H. *Toward a Psychology of Being.* Van Nostrand, Princeton, NJ, 1968.
10. Stevens-Long, J., and Commons, M.L. *Adult Life*, 4th ed. Mayfield Publishing: Mountain View, CA, 1992.
11. Hauser, S. *Adolescents and Their Families.* Free Press: New York, 1991.

5

The Unseen Hand
of Biology I:
Background for Understanding
Mid-Life Sexuality

WHAT DETERMINES OUR PERSONAL
SEXUAL FATE?

Like most other adults, I remain highly interested in this question. My unflagging curiosity about what shapes my sexual adjustment at the various phases of my life is a bit pale, however, when compared to the issue as I confront it daily in clinical practice. There, far less intellectualized, more obviously anxious questions are asked. What is wrong with me (us)? Why am I (are we) having so much difficulty now? Why has this happened to me? Why am I like this? Can you help me?

The main subjects of this and the next chapter are the windows of opportunities—the obstacles and the challenges—presented by the unseen hand of biology. This topic is actually an age-related paradigm for understanding the adult sexual life cycle. When some of our patients ask their anxious questions about why their problems exist and whether we can help them, some of them do not stay around long enough to find out the answers. Some are perhaps too anxious to hear our answers, but others, I have discovered, leave because of us. I want to first address the unpleasant topic of the therapist inadvertently driving the patient away.

The Therapist Rarely Knows the Relevant Information

In my experience, many patients can not or will not tell the therapist everything they know about their sexual problem at the first meeting. However thorough their history taking, therapists should assume that they have not identified all of the relevant factors or, if they have, accurately gauged the relative importance of each of the factors. The crucial issue for the therapist is how to respond to the information that is at our disposal.

To retain our patients, our responses need to reflect an understanding of their lives about which they have not yet spoken. The therapist need not be clairvoyant, only savvy to the incompleteness of any account. We can take a good enough, even an excellent history, but we should not equate covering each relevant topic with having all of the pertinent information. Patient confidence in us is heightened by our responses that indicate to them that we understand that there is more to consider.

Confident Knowledgeable Humility

Both the immediate and lasting outcomes of our therapies are not so unmistakably excellent that we can afford to be arrogant about our usefulness to others. Our frequent disappointing therapy outcomes[1] indicate that either we don't know enough or we cannot significantly influence the relevant factors. This is quite humbling.

The patient's problem is that his sexual life is a jumble. We need to profoundly understand the jumble. Those crucial first hours when we are taking our histories and interviewing the patient are the same hours that the patient is interviewing us, trying to decide if this therapist knows enough, has the right attitude, and can be trusted enough with additional information to be of assistance. Even when we first strike the patient as being the wrong age, gender, race, ethnicity, or orientation, confidence in us is gained by our manner and our knowledge. Our knowledge is not directly displayed; it is reflected in the questions we ask. What the patient cannot know, except perhaps intuitively from our manner, is that our questions reflect unseen paradigms of thought about the causes of problems.

Ignoring the Biology of the Life Cycle

Sexual life, like psychological life in general, is profoundly influenced by continuous processes of change. Some of the changes, like those induced by the menstrual cycle, occur predictably and have a well-known, but often conceptually ignored, cyclicity. Others, like the presence of illness, are abrupt. Most, however, derive from our biological evolution. These are so slow and subtle that they are largely imperceptible. Biology has a hand in the changes that occur in emotional, intellectual, sexual functional, interpersonal, and social spheres and move us in both forward and reverse directions. The rhythmic menstrual changes of sexual desire, arousal, and orgasm, the sudden shifts in our lives from illness or external stresses, and the unseen processes that make up aging make it difficult to be too certain about the exact determinants of sexual problems.

During the 60 or more years of adulthood, we develop through six sexual phases. Each of these carries with it its own set of social and psychological forces, challenges, dilemmas, and problematic outcomes. An entourage of experts tries to solve each phase's sexual problems, but their expertise is limited by many factors. Here are only three:

1. The unwritten social rule that we should not directly discuss, let alone study, sexual matters. It is all right to talk about problematic sex in a medical or psychiatric context; it is generally not acceptable to discuss the healthy possibilities and experience of sexual behavior. As a result we all feel the paradox: We are endlessly curious about sexuality, but remain individually and institutionally silent about its great issues. The facts of sexual life are not secrets—there is nothing here that we as a culture need to keep from one another or lie about to the young. We simply consider how these facts apply to us a matter of privacy.

2. In our rush to be efficient, helpful, and have credentials, we
   think that a sexual problem—for instance, psychogenic erectile dysfunction or women's anorgasmia, is a similar problem
   whenever it occurs in life. The clinical challenges suggest just
   the opposite. Age makes a crucial difference to the nature of
   the problem and the nature of the solution.
3. We resort to simplistic arguments—for instance, it is organic
   versus it is psychogenic—often disguising from ourselves our
   elaborate justification for our particular discipline—psychiatry, psychology, gynecology, urology— rather than appreciating the multiple determinants of this person's current sexual
   fate and realizing that the specific professional may, in the last
   analysis, be helpful with one aspect of the forces that are ad-
   versely affecting the patient.

If I am correct in my measure of "What determines our personal
sexual fate?" this chapter can serve as an antidote for each of these
three erroneous tendencies.

THE SIX PHASES OF ADULT SEXUALITY

Adult life consists of five sequential phases. In addition, a sixth, the
phase of serious physical or psychological illness, may occur at any
time. The lengths of the phases vary enormously from person to person.
They are, nonetheless, developmental stages through which we pass
and to which we often return throughout our lives.

Some individuals manage to pass through these phases in a direct
1 through 6 sequence. Their relatively simple progression is illustrated
by the down arrows in Figure 1. The majority of people, however, have
more complex sequences. Their lives are dynamic—reverberating
through constant readjustments. This is the reason for combining the
down arrows with up arrows. Many individuals, however, enter into
new sexual relationships after relationship breakup or partner death or
have ongoing extramarital relationships. Their pathways are not completely illustrated in Figure 1 but can be imagined by arrows that loop
back to phase 1 to restart the sequence. These looping arrows flow from

One: The Discovery of One's Sexual Characteristics during
                           Uncoupled Adulthood

⇕

Two: The Establishment of the Sexual Equilibrium

⇕

Three: The Preservation of Consensual Sexual Behavior

⇕

Four: The Physiological Declines of Mid-Life

⇕

Five: The Further Declines of Older Age

⇕

Six: The Arrival of Illness

Figure 1. The six stages of adult sexuality.

sexual phases 2, 3, 4, 5, and 6 back to phase 1. When people's lives loop back to phase Discovery of Sexual Characteristics in an Uncoupled Adulthood—they may be at new chronological and maturational ages than when they first discovered their sexual characteristics. For instance, a woman whose sexual characteristics were clear to her as a single 20-year-old finds herself in phase 1 again 40 years later with different sexual characteristics. Many other people form and soon end relationships within a single sexual phase; their pathways involve the sequence 1→2→3→1, which occurs during a period of biologically stable sexual characteristics.

PHASE 1: THE DISCOVERY OF ONE'S
SEXUAL CHARACTERISTICS
DURING UNCOUPLED ADULTHOOD

Six components of sexuality can be defined for any adult. These are the product of biological, social, interpersonal, and psychological development that continuously occurs during childhood, adolescence, and adulthood. The six components fall into two broad categories: sexual identity and sexual function.

Sexual Identity

Sexual Identity is an emotion-, defense-, and conflict-laden issue for as many as 20% of young adults. By the time an individual returns to phase 1 at a later maturational stage of life, the person is likely to have attained a greater degree of self-acceptance of the private and public aspects of sexual identity. What follows is a brief vocabulary and explanation of the components of sexual identity.

1. *Gender identity*—the private sense of self in terms of masculinity and femininity is referred to as our *gender sense* whereas the public aspect of gender identity is referred to as *gender role behavior.*
2. *Orientation*—the private sense of self in terms of the sex (gender) of those who attract us for romantic and sexual purposes is called *erotic orientation*. The sex or gender of those males or females whom we engage in sexual and romantic behaviors is the basis for the term *sexual orientation*.
3. *Intention*—the private sense of self in terms of our preferences for what we want to do with a partner or what we want the partner to do with us during sexual behavior is called *erotic intention*. The behaviors that stem from these mental processes give rise to the the term *sexual intention*.

The final dimension of sexual identity derives from the person's observations about what is happening within him- or herself—who attracts, what sexually excites, and how masturbation and partner sex is arranged. Based on these observations the person labels the self with one or more of these terms: *normal, conventional, ordinary, unusual, transvestite, transsexual, homosexual, heterosexual, bisexual, gay, lesbian, asexual, pedophilic, sadistic, masochistic, exhibitionistic, voyeuristic,* or *weird.* Although some of these words only describe one component of sexual identity—that is, of the gender identity, orientation, or intention—they are commonly used to convey the most problematic component of sexual identity. These identity labels have enormous psychological and social significance. They help clinicians to understand what some people mean when they tell us that although they are homoerotic and behave homosexually, they are "not gay." They mean, we can now see, that the private and behavioral aspects of their orientation are homosexual but their personal, social, and political identifications are not with the gay community. There are many homosexual men and women who do not outwardly or inwardly identify with gay and lesbian communities.

During adolescence and later, individuals may have dramatic struggles as their sexual identity unfolds within them. They confront the fact that categories exist in culture for how they are as a sexual person. They may reject, accept, or feel ambivalently about these categories, but their sexual psychologies cannot be understood without knowing how they view themselves and their behaviors. For the majority of people who simply sense themselves as "normal," however, sexual identity is a mere concept that does not seem personally relevant. These individuals often come to be embroiled in other important sexual issues.

Sexual Function

Regardless of the particular components of our sexual identity we have three separate physiological capacities:

1. Desire, which was discussed in the last chapter
2. Arousal, which is a bodywide pleasant physiological process in which changes in blood flow, attention and sensual concentration, respiration, and heart rate build to a level of intensity that triggers the most dramatic aspect of sexual function

3. Orgasm, which is the reflex sequence that returns the body to its prearousal state by way of a brief, intensely pleasurable, fatiguing event

Young single adults exist at their *biological* peak of sexual intensity and efficiency. Their sensory nervous systems work exquisitely, arousal may occur spontaneously both during the day and during the night, and orgasmic attainment, duration, intensity, and repeatability are measurably superior than decades later in life. Whether young adults realize their biological potentials, however, depends on many nonbiological factors. Despite their biological advantage, many single young adults do not have their best sexual experiences during phase 1. Men frequently cannot modulate their sexual excitement and consequently ejaculate too soon to provide their partners with much sensual abandonment or intercourse experience. Women may be so occupied with pleasing their partners that they find that their arousal does not intensify to orgasm. Less often, young men may not be able to ejaculate and young adult women experience painful intercourse. Even when people are not sexually dysfunctional in this phase, their sexual encounters often contain a mixture of pleasant anticipation, pleasant sensations, fear, and inhibition. The mixture makes some people seem comfortable and others nervous. Extreme discomfort with partner sexual expression is not rare, moderate discomfort is far more common, and slight anxiety about sexual behavior is ordinary—even when a person returns to phase 1 after long existing sexual confidence at another stage.

Although the psychoanalytically influenced mental health establishment has long taught that early life parent–child difficulties are the source of young adult sexual dysfunctions, we should keep an open mind. Everyone's sexual life must not be equally vulnerable to developmental difficulties. We do not know what has to happen for a young person to develop sexual comfort. Nor do we know what guarantees the failure to develop sexual function abilities. Some people function well sexually despite horrendous backgrounds and the presence of psychiatric diagnoses. We should not be glib in our explanations.

Given our inability to conceptualize what is needed for sexual adequacy, it is safer to think of sexual comfort, pleasure, and competence as *potentials* that many people do not attain during their first experience with phase 1. Sexual health may await later developmental processes.

In phase 1, each person, whether aged 20 or 60, has a personal display of his or her gender identity, orientation, intention, desire, arousal, and orgasm characteristics. What a person is (identity) and can experience sexually (function) differs broadly from person to person. Whatever they consist of, the six component characteristics are part of the subtle negotiation processes that lead to or prevent phase 2.

PHASE 2: THE ESTABLISHMENT OF THE SEXUAL EQUILIBRIUM

General Schema of the Sexual Equilibrium

When two people establish couplehood for sexual and other purposes, a new phase is initiated. Their new individual sexual fates may be quickly determined by three subtle steps:

1. The six sexual components of each person interact and create an equilibrium
2. The partners' specific component characteristics are regarded in some private manner
3. The partners perceive and emotionally react to how each is regarded

When a person perceives positive regard from the partner, his or her motivation to repeat sexual behavior increases; relaxation, spontaneity, and personal sensual abandonment increase during sex; positive attitudes toward the self and partner are stabilized, partner sexual behavior increases in frequency, private masturbation decreases; and the world of other partners becomes far less alluring.

When a person perceives negative regard from the partner, his or her motivation to repeat sexual behavior decreases; anxiety about and inhibition during sex increases; negative attitudes toward the self and hostility toward the partner occur; partner sexual behavior declines in frequency; private masturbation increases; and thoughts of having sex with another person increase.

The crucial end product of the three subtle steps is *emotional satisfaction*.[2] Mutual emotional satisfaction from sex is the major determinant of frequently recurring sexual behavior within a couple.

What Is Balanced within the Sexual Equilibrium?

Although these processes subtly and quickly occur within each new couple, the resulting emotional satisfaction that occurs is not static. One or more of each person's sexual function component characteristics may change, the way they are regarded may change, and the perception of that regard may become more or less acute. All of these dynamic variables create an ever-changing balance, a sexual equilibrium, that explains why sexual behavior with the same partner is not entirely predictable. The term *equilibrium* implies a balance of component and attitudinal forces that continually readjusts producing a slightly different outcome each time.

Examples of Influence of Regard

- *Two young sex-loving men who ejaculate within 30 seconds of intercourse, that is, they possess the same component characteristic.* One has a partner who is annoyed at her deprivation and, after kindly masking her disappointment for several months, suggests to her eager lover that they should read a book about premature ejaculation. Now more anxiously aware of her wish to experience orgasm during intercourse with him, his concern with the timing of his orgasm preoccupies him during sex. He begins to appear nervous to her during sex. He becomes an even less satisfying lover because he no longer can sensually abandon himself and his perfunctory manner inhibits her more than when he was just ejaculating quickly. Despite her ability to attain orgasm by hand or mouth stimulation, their sexual behaviors together become much less frequent.

  The second man continues to think of his partner as happy with him. She tells him how much she enjoys his orgasmic sounds and release and, when he asks if she attained orgasm during intercourse, she says "no" but indicates only that what he does by hand or mouth is fine. He perceives that she likes sex even when she does not attain orgasm in any way. He thinks of himself as a good-enough lover. Their sexual frequency continues to be high, both are happy, and he gradually attains more ejaculatory control.

- *Two women who attain orgasm readily only through manual genital stimulation, that is, they have the same component characteristic.* One has a partner who feels cheated by her "inhibition." He clearly explains himself to her, thinking that she needs some help because he so much desires to bring her to orgasm during intercourse. She tries harder, is still unable to let herself go, and becomes more nervous during sex. She fears that she will be abandoned by him because he has been with others who had orgasms during intercourse. Sex gradually becomes infrequent.

  The second woman's partner is delighted by her arousal, he does not think of her vagina as a proving ground for his masculinity. He loves her movement from high level of arousal to orgasm and tells her so repeatedly. Their equilibrium continues to generate frequent sexual behavior.

Example of the Influence of Differences in a Component Characteristic

- *Two readily orgasmic 25-year-old women who feel sexual drive premenstrually.* One has sex with her partner twice monthly because his drive becomes distracting about every two weeks and he then initiates sex. He enjoys sex but rarely feels urgent about it. She is emotionally and physically satisfied. She initiates sex occasionally—usually premenstrually.

  The other woman behaves sexually with her partner twice weekly because that is about how often he initiates. He loves sex and feels that his life will deteriorate if he does not make love several times a week. She is emotionally and physically satisfied during sex. She initiates sex occasionally—usually premenstrually.

It takes a number of sexual experiences together for a new couple to get a sense of the sexual potential of their new entity. The early sexual experiences may be more nervous than relaxed, more accommodating than sensual, more polite than spontaneous. But after a while, the couple settles into something familiar and unique. Their sexual equilibrium is balanced by both component interaction and regard. Regard is an attitude that has both private and shared features. Individuals keep many of their attitudes about the sexual characteristics of their partners private—for very good reasons. Discovering some of them causes our partners to lose their capacity for sensual abandonment, pushes them in the direction of excessive self-consciousness during sexual behavior, and motivates them to avoid sexual behavior.

The key accomplishment in a couple's equilibrium is not orgasm, mutual orgasm, orgasm during intercourse, or multiple orgasms during 20 minutes of intercourse, however nice all of this sounds. Rather, it is emotional satisfaction, which more reliably shapes the frequency of sexual behavior. The formation and early evolution of the sexual equilibrium mold the sexual patterns of the new couple and announce to each person the range of experiences that can be expected within the new social entity. They may be optimistic about their sexual future together, they may think they have a good-enough, if not great, sex life, but their sexual fate has not been determined in any final developmental sense— unless the sexual equilibrium is so unsatisfying to one or both partners that sexual behavior disappears.

PHASE 3: THE PRESERVATION OF CONSENSUAL SEXUAL BEHAVIOR

Many couples initially maintain a mutually satisfactory sexual equilibrium, yet their sexual lives dwindle in frequency, develop arousal and orgasm dysfunctions, and cease to be emotionally satisfying. Some of this results from their failure as a couple to privately fully consent to sexual behavior. This is an important subtlety; it easily can get lost when the details of a couple's lives are heard. There are two larger factors that organize the explanation for the deterioration of the quality of sexual life after a satisfactory sexual equilibrium has been established. Each is a developmental challenge shared by the partners.

1. *Valuing the importance of sexual behavior.* People either genuinely do not understand or else they act as though they do not understand the important roles sexual behavior can play in our lives. For a couple's sexual life to survive, it is vital that both individuals jointly value their sexual behavior together. Men and women, regardless of orientation, need to reflect on four important nonreproductive reasons for making love.

   - Lovemaking confirms, stabilizes, and enables personal celebration of one's sexual identity.
   - Lovemaking is widely understood as one of life's great dependable sources of pleasure; it is what many consider to be part of their strategy for the pursuit of happiness.
   - Lovemaking provides a wordless affirmation of the bond to the partner.
   - Lovemaking can be emotional tonic for minor distress—it can eradicate annoyance, sadness, anxiety, insomnia, horniness, and the like.

2. *Respecting the need to manage anger and disappointment well.* It is inevitable that people will be disappointed and angry with one another. Young women's desire, arousal, orgasm, and emotional satisfaction are generally more responsive to resentment and disappointment than are young men's, but this does not mean that men are exempt. As people get older, these sex differences tend to dissipate. Sexual desire, arousal, and emotional satisfaction can deteriorate quickly in both sexes when disappointment and resentment remain unsuccessfully processed. Although individuals participate in sex, their anger and disappointment keep them from doing so with any interest, that is, they do not fully privately consent to sexual behavior.

   Because men's sexual drives generally exceed women's, men carry more resentment over not having sex than do women. This is part of the background noise in many men's awareness: Regardless of why sex becomes infrequent, many men feel resentment that it is infrequent. One of the strongest motivations for discussing a new interpersonal problem for the couple is to be able to return to the diverse pleasures of love-making. Preservation of sexual life together requires making a commitment to quickly attempt to repair the inevitable rifts that arise as two people try to harmonize their individual lives. No couple who has sexually survived the previous phase can escape from the two weighty challenges of phase 3. To preserve sexual health the couple has to act as though they know that sex is important and they have to deal effectively with their disagreements and disappointments. If they do this well, one would hope that their sexual fate would continue to be positive, but phase 4 is coming.

REFERENCES

1. Segraves, R.T., and Althof, S.E. Psychotherapy and pharmacotherapy. In: J. Gorman (ed.), *Treatments That Work*. Oxford University Press: London, in press.
2. Levine, S.B. *Sexual Life:A Clinician's Guide*. Plenum: New York, 1992, Chapter 4.

6

The Unseen Hand of Biology II: The Fifties and Beyond

PHASE 4: PHYSIOLOGICAL DECLINES OF MIDDLE AGE

Variation is the rule in all biological matters. Some of the processes that are described here as occuring in the years 50–60 show up for some individuals in their 40s and even, rarely, in the late 30s. For others, primarily men, the events are delayed until the next decade. In reading about phase #4, it is important not to confuse the topic of the chapter--the expectable *physiological* decline--with the topics of love and psychological intimacy. It is ironic that many people finally are able to consistently act in a loving fashion and speak and listen intimately only when their bodies are gradually losing their previous smoothly functioning sexual capacities.

Women

Sexual Phenomenology

Over 1 million American women enter menopause annually.[1] Those who are not already clearly heading into menopause by their 50th birthday will soon begin to notice physiological changes that will affect their sexual lives during this decade. The hallmark explanation of menopause is estrogen deficiency. The many physiological consequences of this biologically predictable loss of estrogen are well described in the medical and lay literature. The multiple sexual effects on the reproductive tract and on other organ systems are far less well known, however. These effects are difficult to separate from the inexorable aging process.[2] Patients, and occasionally physicians, sometimes assume that all of the menopause-related changes of their sexuality are reversible with hormone replacement therapy. The evidence for this, however, is neither clear nor extensive.[3] Estrogen alone or combinations of estrogen with progesterone or with androgen may slow some of these changes, but they do not entirely stop the early decline of the sexual response system.

It is not known with certainty how many women of each year of age—for instance, 46, 47, 48, 49, 50—have noticed one or more of the items on the following list. Some studies have suggested that up to 50% of women[4] notice these changes as they naturally enter into menopause.[5] The percentage of women noticing these changes may be considerably higher in clinics specializing in menopausal concerns. Presumably some groups of women experience these changes less frequently.

1. Slowness of vaginal lubrication
2. Diminished volume of vaginal lubrication, occasionally to the point of painful intercourse for the woman or man
3. Less erotic response to vulvar, clitoral, breast, and nipple stimulation
4. More difficulty focusing on the tactile sensations that previously efficiently created a state of sexual arousal
5. Diminished drive or an increased freedom from the feeling that sex with partner or masturbation is necessary to restore comfort
6. Fewer sexual fantasies and preoccupations

These are the biology-based sexual changes of the perimenopausal and early menopausal years. Most are present well before the last menstrual period. It is important to emphasize the *biological* basis of these changes because women themselves tend to explain the earliest manifestations as being related to social or psychological factors. Psychological factors within the sexual equilibrium come into play, as they always do, during the perimenopausal–menopausal phase and add to the variability of sexual experience from woman to woman.

The efficiency of sexual behavior diminishes during this phase. In terms of the three components of sexual function—desire, arousal, and orgasm, orgasmic capacity remains the least affected during the early postmenopausal years, but even some of its physiological characteristics may change. The sensations of genital stimulation by hand, mouth, penis, or vibrator may be noticably different or more difficult to attain. The loss of sexual efficiency is not a topic, however, women and their doctors—of either sex—are generally at ease discussing. These sexual changes add to women's sense that they are getting old. "Getting old" often communicates feeling different in their bodies, noticing changing body contours, a diminished sense of sexual attractiveness and confidence, and becoming relatively invisible to the roving eyes of men.[6]

It is reasonable to ask about the women of this phase who do not report or are not sexually affected by this biological process. Three explanations have already been mentioned: (1) Biological changes are always variable in their expression, both as to when and to what degree they occur; (2) women are reticient to discuss the topic with physicians; (3) this topic has not been extensively researched and the research that has been done is not widely known.

Two additional explanations make the sexual changes of this phase not particularly significant to certain women: (5) Many women's sexual lives have not survived the developmental challenges posed by earlier phases. A combination of never-mastered childhood sexual anxieties (phase 1), adjustment problems within their sexual equilibrium (phase 2), and failure to adequately negotiate the nonsexual challenges of couplehood (phase 3) have long before created various forms of sexual avoidance or male-oriented sexual servicing that basically are a decathexis of personal sexual life. For these women, the loss of personal sexual efficiency is irrelevant. (5) Other more compelling life problems—such as physical illness in the family, behavioral troubles with a child, or financial difficulties—make the sexual changes of the perimenopausal period hardly worthy of mention. Thus, by the fourth phase of sexual life, some women have long ago given up on the aspiration to have a wonderful sexual life. These women find relief in their loss of sexual feelings and capacities and hide behind the belief that "I'm too old for that now."

Endocrine Physiology

The endocrinological basis for menopause is not a topic that is very well understood. An appreciation of its complexity begins with an awareness that three broad types of menopause are recognized. Although each type is characterized by estrogen deficiency, the pathways to this physiological state differ.[7]

1. *Natural*
2. *Premature*—definitions vary between less than 40 and less than 45 years of age for this apparently normal occurrence. Cigarette smoking may play a role in the genesis of premature menopause.[8]
3. *Artificial*—induced by surgery, illness, medication, radiation[9]

In natural menopause, the process is gradual and may occur over as much as a decade or more before the last menstrual period.[10] Estradiol and progesterone gradually diminish and follicle-stimulating hormone levels (FSH) increase. Ovarian granulosa cell production of inhibin, a hormone that limits the production of FSH, slowly diminishes. As a consequence, FSH levels remain high. Levels above 40 IU\liter are the accepted standard indication of ovarian failure.

Between the phase of regular menstruation and menopause, ovarian production rates for individual hormones diminish to differing degrees. Estradiol production diminishes by approximately 85%, estrone by approximately 58% (estrone is the weaker estrogen which menopausal women convert in small amounts to estradiol). Ovarian production rates of the androgens diminish less than the estrogens. The androstenedione rates fall approximately 67% while testosterone production diminishes only approximately 29%. Progesterone diminishes 99%. Estrogen levels can be quite variable from woman to woman because the ovaries may still periodically secrete estrogens in the first few years after the last menses.[11]

Many consider menopause to result not only from a relative ovarian failure but also from changes in the pituitary gland. Luetinizing hormone (LH) continues to stimulate the ovarian stroma's production of testosterone, but not as efficiently. Adrenal cortical androgens, such as dehydroepiandrosterone (DHAS), which are stimulated by ACTH, also reach a low point around the menopause. DHAS is the most abundant androgen in circulation. It declines throughout adulthood until menopause when it stabilizes.

Women who undergo hysterectomy but retain their ovaries enter menopause on average 4 years earlier than those with a natural menopause. Blood flow to the ovaries is often diminished following hysterectomy. This may be part of the explanation for the earlier menopause of these women. In contrast, when both ovaries are removed the symptoms of estrogen and androgen deficiency are more abrupt and severe. LH and FSH reach maximum concentration within 1 year, which is earlier than for those with natural menopause. These pituitary hormone levels remain high for the next 20 years in contrast to women with a natural menopause whose LH and FSH levels decline with age. Oophorectomized women have a decline in adrenal cortical androgen secretion as well. Women who undergo a unilateral oophorectomy may have irregular menstrual cycles earlier in life than those who keep both ovaries.

Menopause induced by ovarian disease, by medications for illnesses such as lupus or cancer, or by radiation are complicated by the underlying conditions and therefore are more difficult to characterize physiologically. Certain systemic illnesses, such as chronic obstructive pulmonary disease, create hypoxia, which in turn may lead to lower testosterone levels and diminished ovarian function.

Sexual Anatomical, Physiological, and Behavioral Changes

However it comes about, menopause affects sexual capacity. The major underlying consequence of ovarian failure is a decrease in pelvic blood flow. Pubic hair becomes thinner and coarser. The labia majora shrink, as do the labia minora and clitoris. Progressively fewer women exhibit expansion and color changes of the labia as they pass into their 60s.[12] The tumescent responses of the clitoris occur in only about 20% of women over age 50. The vagina bears the most significant impact of the menopause. Its changes are more apparent than those of the external genital structures. Its surface flattens, losing its rough, ridged appearance. The surface initially thins to just a few cell layers, making capillaries visible, but with further atrophy the surface becomes smooth, shiny, and pale. The depth decreases, and the walls lose their elasticity because fibrous connective tissue replaces muscle cells. The biochemical environment becomes less acidic, which creates a shift in vaginal flora. The uterus gradually returns to its prepubertal size. The dramatic decrease (approximately 60%) in blood flow to the vulva and vaginal areas and the histological effects of this process explain the slower and less copious vaginal lubrication. Orgasmic contractions of the vagina still occur at age 60 but contraction of the rectum does not seem to occur as it does in premenopausal women. Several common symptoms of this phase seem to be related to these changes: dyspareunia, postintercourse spotting, postintercourse urinary tract infections, vaginitis, and vulvadynia.

Rates of masturbation and of marital sexual behavior decline in the perimenopausal and menopausal years. Women evidence significantly more sexual disinterest and absence of sex than men at the same age range. This pattern is far more dramatic in the middle years than earlier.[13] In the 1970s, studies of the sexual patterns of menopausal women found that sexual changes were almost entirely explained by their partners' diminishing interest, ability, health, or availability. This conclusion no longer seems tenable.[14]

Hallström carefully looked at the question of women's sexual changes with a physically healthy large sample and demonstrated that: (1) the climacteric brought reduction in sexual interest, capacity for orgasm, and coital frequency and (2) this was not simply a response to the husbands' declining interest.[15] McCoy and Davidson confirmed these findings in a prospective study and demonstrated that the largest decline in sexual behavior occurred in the 12–24 months prior to the last menses.[16]

It is now apparent that the sexual changes of this phase have previously been underemphasized. Much of the literature for the lay public minimizes the sexual consequences of the menopause, except to suggest they are correctable with estrogen and sex counseling.[17,18]

The Hormonal Fix of Menopausal Sexual Deficits?

Fixing the sexual deficits of this phase is not high on most physicians' minds. Physicians and their patients often do not discuss the sexual consequences of menopause. The indications for hormone replacement therapy revolve around issues such as quickly stopping the bothersome dysfunctions of thermoregulation, and the delaying of osteoporosis and heart disease, when they weigh the pros and cons of prescribing hormone replacement therapy. When sexual deficits are brought up, however, physicians have an understandable therapeutic desire to provide hormones to rejuvenate sexual interest and responsivity. A controlled study has shown that the use of estrogens positively correlates with most parameters of sexual function.[19] Correlations are not the same as clinically adequate responses, however. Much clinical experience and many studies suggest that estrogens alone do not correct most of the sexual deficits in menopausal women. This is particularly true of natural estrogens such as conjugated equine estrogens, including the most widely prescribed Premarin. Estrogens may, however, initially help many women to generally and sexually feel considerably better.[20]

Androgens are often quoted as the hormone group that creates sexual drive in both sexes, but how this is physiologically accomplished is a mystery. Women have three sources of androgens: (1) the ovaries, (2) the adrenals, and (3) the peripheral conversion of other sex steroids to testosterone in adipose tissue, muscle, and skin. Menstruating women generate about 7 mg of testosterone a month from three sources: 25% from the ovaries, 25% from the adrenals, and 50% from peripheral conversion.[21] Androgens circulate both bound to carrier proteins and in a free or unbound state. Higher levels of estrogen lessen the binding of androgens. Sexual drive may be a result of androgen effects within the brain as well as many other places in the body. Receptors for sex steroids exist in many tissues including the breast, vagina, skin, vulva, urethra, bladder trigone, uterus, oviducts, blood vessels, pituitary, hypothalamus, limbic forebrain, and cortex. Although androgens usually decline in the natural menopause, a minority of women may actually have more for several years. They may have differing sources of androgen—more from peripheral conversion, less from the ovarian stroma. When women's menopausal sexual symptoms are treated with testosterone, the amounts given are usually far greater than 7 mg/month. The physiology of drive must be far more refined and complex than the therapeutic approach of providing supranormal levels of this hormone. The highest doses of androgens are those given by injection; when androgens are given in pill form, poor absorption and first-pass hepatic metabolism limit serum levels. Hormones are regulated by feedback mechanisms so that if exogenous testosterone is given, endogenous production may decline. In addition, the initial high-dose effects of androgens do not necessarily continue as the supranormal levels are maintained.[22] Women's sexual drive is not merely manipulatable by administration of androgens. It is clear that an unknown complexity remains to be elucidated.

Men in their 50s often experience a decreased sex drive without a dramatic decrement in their androgen production. Their endocrine milieu is less complex than women's. This raises the possibility that the sexual drive deficits are part of a larger physiological process (aging) that is measured by endocrine changes, loss of cellular receptors for androgen, loss of enzymatic activity that converts testosterone into a form that can be used within the cytoplasm or nucleus of cells, and unknown features. Menopause per se may be only a small and relatively unimportant part of the explanation. It is far more sobering to think that sexual drive deficits are part of the genetic programming of human beings and have multiple complex bodywide determinants involving subcellular, cellular, tissue, and organ system changes.

The strongest evidence that androgen replacement can help with the sexual symptoms of menopause is seen in 3-month placebo-controlled studies of ovariectomized women whose treatment protocol began 4 months after surgical menopause. Only those with testosterone or estrogen–testosterone injections improved sexually; those on placebo or estrogen alone did not.[23] Left unanswered is the question of how long testosterone can sustain the sexual interest of these women. The data are far less clear that administration of androgens to women with a natural menopause reverses their new sexual deficits. The good results are largely anecdotal.[24] Typically, they occur after the woman has not responded to therapy with estrogen alone; the use of androgens is often the next recommended step.[25] A few controlled studies have suggested a modest effect, but the issues of sample selection, differences in sex steroids used and their dosages, the duration of the positive results, and means of assessing sexual effects point to the need for additional careful study.[26]

Estrogens are used widely now for four reasons:

1. Their dramatic ameliorative effects on hot flashes and flushes
2. Their long-term effects on delaying the onset of heart disease
3. Their slowing of the rate of osteoporosis
4. Their impact on insufficient vaginal lubrication, pain on intercourse, intolerance to genital touch[27]

The results of studies of the effect of estrogen replacement on lubrication adequacy generally consistently point toward improvement. All preparations of estrogens are able to help in this way. How long this effect lasts and what percentage of sexually active women still need external lubricants are not clear, however. Although studies generally cover 6 months or less, one 2-year study demonstrated continual improvement over the study period.[28] Once vaginal lubrication is restored, however, the issue for the individual woman remains her level of sexual interest. When estrogens are perceived to have helped with a diminished sexual drive, the effects are thought either to be indirect by helping with other matters that increase the sense of well-being,[29] to be slight, to affect only some women, [19] or to be related to the specific compound used. None of five studies using conjugated equine estrogens has demonstrated any improvement in sexual interest.[30] Modern combination preparations (for those with a uterus) contain progestins, which throughout menstruating life have been thought to diminish sexual drive.

Here is another reason for caution. Using sophisticated statistical analyses, a carefully done community-based study of middle-aged women not on hormone replacement failed to demonstrate any contribution of either serum estrogens or androgens to carefully defined parameters of sexual adjustment.[31]

The most encouraging information about sexual function in this age group has confirmed an older clinical impression: In a study of 52 women between ages 50 and 67, those who had intercourse at least 3 times a month had less vaginal atrophy than those who had intercourse less than 10 times a year.[32] Similarly, in a study of perimenopausal women, weekly intercourse was associated with less urogenital atrophy.[33]

Clinicians need to keep one additional observation in mind when hormone replacement therapy (HRT) is offered as the solution to menopausal sexual deficits. The acceptance rate of HRT in studies done by academic investigators is high—approximately 80% of women maintain their treatment during the study protocols. In community studies of the administration of HRT for menopausal symptoms, however, the average woman begun on HRT changes preparations 2.2 times. After 3 years, three quarters of women are no longer on HRT.[34] The reasons for this include: wishing to no longer have periods (not all HRT regimens create menses); dislike of premenstrual-like discomfort; episodes of breakthrough bleeding that require a workup for uterine cancer; fear of breast or uterine cancer; and the wish to live naturally. A study of

British physicians begun on HRT found that 50% were taking them after several years.[35] Even among women who are the among the most
highly informed about the short- and long-term benefits of HRT, the
drop out rate is high. So there are two reasons to be less than optimistic
about HRT as the solution to the problem of menopausal sexual deficits: It is not clear to what extent and for what duration they actually reverse the array of sexual deficits and most women will not persist in
using HRT.

Case Three: Perimenopausal Sexual Deficits that Persisted

A 56-year-old still regularly menstruating teacher came to see me
3 years ago because of sexual complaints: decreased breast and genital
sensations, inability to concentrate and become aroused during sex, occasional dysesthesias genitally. She had been to four physicians—an
internist, two gynecologists, and a neurologist—who looked for various explanations of her difficulty but could provide none. In the process, a syrinx in her cervical–thoracic cord was found, making her very
anxious about the possibility of becoming paralyzed. Initially she
thought this was the reason for her breast insensitivity, but two neurolo-
gists said that they considered her spinal cord lesion to be only an inci-
dental finding. She had loved her sexual life and felt deeply distressed
by its dramatic decline in the last several years.

She proudly told me of her continuing menstruation—a genetic
trait apparently as each of her sisters menstruated until almost age 60.
With much encouragement from me, she asked several of them about
whether they experienced changes in their sexual functioning when
they were her age. They said that they did not think so but were obviously embarrassed. I told her that I was sorry to say that many physicians, including gynecologists, either did not seem to know about the
sexual impact of the perimenopausal years or were too uncomfortable
to discuss it. This was only one of the issues she brought to me: The major problem was her sense of being overwhelmed by the difficulties that
she was experiencing on all fronts—her frail ancient mother who lived
with her, her daughter's depression, her son's career difficulties, the demands at work, and her husband's slowly deteriorating health. She felt

that she could not take much more of whatever was happening. Although complaining of a host of depressive symptoms, she was deeply opposed to the idea of taking medication. As we began to talk about her life in more detail, she told me of her enduring sense of being beleaguered by problems. "I came from a family that could not afford to educate me for my actual ambitions. We had a 6-week-old son who died of crib death. My mother has lived with me for over 14 years. Now that she is immobile, I constantly worry that she will fall."

She was quite productive and managed to excel at work and at her extra teaching job; she recognized that she gravitated to increasing her burdens. She was intense and driven and always feared not getting her work done or not doing it well.

These days I see her periodically when she is in need of talking through some profound threatening change in her life. This time it is her husband's impending lung surgery. She looks exhausted.

Thanks for seeing me on such short notice. I had to talk to you. There is nowhere else I can turn. Ted won't allow me to tell anyone—the children, my sisters, my friends—about the recommendation for surgery. The doctor said it was not an emergency but he thinks that it should be done within the next few months. He just keeps on working, traveling, and making out to his colleagues that he is just fine. Meantime, he looks terrible. What will happen if he dies? I don't think that I can survive. [She cries.]

Ted makes this tough situation so much tougher. You are so loyal to his wishes in this regard. When will he tell the kids?

He says about a week before the surgery and first he has to decide when he will have it based on what is happening at work. Ted thinks that the more people who know about this, the more likely it is that he will be asked all sorts of questions about this private matter. He has always kept me out of his health issues. I've had big arguments over the years because he won't let me talk to his doctors. He reminds me that it is his body and he has a right to manage it his way.

Well, he has been consistent. It would make me angry at him, if I were you. Are you resentful that he restricts you from your sisters?

I am angry, but I'm more worried. What can I do? That's why I came to see you—I felt I was going to explode.

Comment: Her sexual life has not improved over 3 years, but her husband's deterioration has moved it down on her problem priority list. They did have a few sexual experiences on minivacations during which she felt more aroused, but she has never been orgasmic since this problem with erotic sensations arrived. Two varieties of hormone replacement have not ameliorated the situation. Her gynecologist had hoped that hormone replacement would improve her mood but this has not occurred.

Men

Sexual Phenomenology

As male testosterone levels do not diminish in the same predictable manner as do estrogens, it seems incorrect to refer to the sexual decline of the 50s as the male menopause. But the concept of this analogous physiological state lingers in our public and medical thinking. This is simply because many men in their 50s notice that they are not sexually like they were in their 40s. Physicians who think they have discovered various treatments for the declining sexual capacities of this age tend to favor the term *male menopause.*

The big differences between the 40s and 50s are a decline in sexual drive and a loss of erectile security. Drive declines are noticed earlier in the decade, unreliability of erections later. Terms like erectile security and erectile unreliability refer to difficulties attaining full tumescence, maintaining firm erections long enough to complete intercourse, and occasionally not erecting at all during sexual behavior. Most physically healthy men in their 50s are potent. But the use of the term potent increasingly connotes a subtlety. With time potency becomes a matter of degree—no longer can men depend on having an absolute reliable, rigid, long-enough erection until orgasm. Some men in this decade, however, have erectile dysfunction.

The most common age at which men seek help for impotence from urologists is the late 50s. They usually have had the problem for about 2 years before seeking assistance. An unusually carefully done study of physically, psychologically, and maritally healthy men has demonstrated a significant decline in the frequency and duration of nocturnal erections between ages 45–54 and 55–65.[36] This study makes clear that the male sexual system is declining. The decline is severe enough to create a significant degree of erectile unreliability in up to 30% of 60-year-olds.[37] This 30% figure is a summary of many studies performed over several decades. Just as the more recent studies of menopausal sexuality are demonstrating higher degrees of sexual impairment, so the more current studies of men, using more sophisticated methods, are revealing larger percentages of men with compromised potency. A study of impotence among 1290 men between the ages of 40 and 70, for instance, found that 10% were completely, 25% moderately, and 17% minimally impaired.[38] This study generated correlational evidence that the risk factors for moderate and complete impairment were the same factors that put men at risk for atherosclerotic heart disease: smoking, hypertension, obesity, abnormal lipids, and diabetes. Correlational studies, of course, cannot establish the cause of phenomena.

The good biological news in this phase is that some men are able to attain good ejaculatory control for the first time in their lives. Because ejaculation is accomplished less efficiently, both the men and their partners may conclude that they have become better lovers. In a more subtle fashion, this sexual attainment may actually be associated with less intense penile sensations during early intercourse. The other encouraging factor is that even though erections may not be as reliably firm, they are good enough to enable intercourse. Perhaps the diminished turgidity decreases vaginal friction and enables a lesser degree of lubrication to be sufficient.

A recent important study of sexual behavior in the United States, which applied the most ideal sampling methods to ascertain the prevalence of sexual dysfunctions of men and women between the ages 18 and 59, produced a slightly different impression. The prevalence of premature ejaculation was reported to be relatively stable throughout this period. This is not the impression one gets from patient care. The prevalence of men who have had difficulties with maintaining erections

for at least several months during the previous year increased significantly each 5 year interval.[39]

The Causes of Erectile Dysfunction during the 50s

Urologists are now leading the charge to define the causes of erectile problems and to find new effective treatments. They define health
during this decade to include reliable erectile function. If men are not
potent, the urologist looks for the disease that explains the dysfunction.
Here is a common classification of the causes: vascular disease,
medication-induced, endocrinopathy, traumatic injury, systemic
chronic illness, depression. During the last decade, urologists have
demonstrated a wide variety of penile physiological abnormalities in
this age group. Unfortunately, they have rarely taken the scientific care
to separate age effects from disease effects. What is striking epidemiol-
ogically about the burgeoning data, however, is that erectile dysfunction
is far more prevalent in those with physical diseases such as hypertension, diabetes, and atherosclerosis than in men without these conditions.
This has been demonstrated numerous times in various population
groups. The repeated finding tends to implicate the disease itself in
causing the problem. Caution is in order, however. A most important observation was made in Schiavi and colleague's study of healthy men
taking no medication: nocturnal erections and sexual erections with
partners diminish dramatically in men between 55 and 64 when compared with men a decade younger.[36] Even in health—happily married,
on no medication, no history of illness, no evidence of illness on physical and laboratory examination—many men in their late 50s have unreliable erections—that is, sometimes adequate, sometimes not, and some
are unable to have intercourse. Well, cynics on one side may argue that
even in these healthy men, penile disease may have been present that
was too subtle to detect with the thorough but noninvasive diagnostic
tests performed. Cynics on the other side might argue that the effects on
the penis are a condition but not a disease—more like presbyopia that
suddenly strikes people in their mid-40s. The genetic program for the
human is to have a diminishing potency beginning in this decade. "Conditions" may cause impairment but they are not related to a disease. For
many people, the only question is, "Can something be done about this
without unacceptable side effects?" Mere semantic debate over words

like *presbyopia*, *presbycusia* and, *presbyrectia* is of little interest. The person still cannot read well, hear well, or count on his penis— whatever name is applied to the condition. It is not just biology and philosophy; it is about creating expectations that cannot be realized or inducing new problems that cannot be immediately perceived.[40] The body's systems have differing longevities. In our arrogant optimism, we refuse to recognize the unwinding of biological potential as normal; we make it into disease and look for causes both personally ("It's because I was unfaithful early in my marriage that I'm being punished now") and medically ("Cigarette smoking increases the risk of impotence"). For others who just want to keep their potency a few decades longer, the only issues are effectiveness and safety. The answers to the question, "Are the new treatments effective and safe?" increasingly seem to be an acceptable "yes." As medicine progresses further, there is reason to believe that more men and couples will be interested in what can be done for the aging sexual system—diseased or not.

Several lines of investigation are converging on the hypothesis that the underlying common pathway of impotence of aging and of various vascular diseases is hypoxia within the corpora cavernosa. The normal architecture of these erectile bodies in youth contains approximately 50% smooth muscle. As men age, the percentage of collagen increases and the amount of functional smooth muscle tissue decreases significantly.[41] Cavernosal smooth muscle relaxation is the key intracorporal physiological event leading to erection. It is brought about by several converging pathways. The best known is the nitric oxide (NO) mechanism. NO is produced in the endothelial cells by NO synthetase and by the stimulation of nonadrenergic noncholinergic nerves. NO diffuses into the smooth muscle where it stimulates the production of cyclic guanosine monophosphate (cGMP) which causes vasodilation.[42] Erection is the physiological result of vasodilation of the arterioles leading to the sinusoids and of the smooth muscles within the cavernosal sinusoids. Hypoxia from any cause decreases the production of NO and increases the production of enzymes that generate collagen. Aging in most tissues studied throughout the body generates an increased production of collagen. Penile tissue has an extremely low oxygen tension during the flaccid state. An appealing current theory is that nocturnal erections maintain NO synthetase levels by periodically increasing penile blood flow and preventing hypoxia. Anything that limits oxygenation of the penis—that is, vascular insufficiencies or diminished nocturnal erections—may shift the biochemistry of the penis in a direction that generates the conversion of smooth muscle to fibroblastic tissue and thereby generates erectile unreliability and eventually impotence.[43]

In fact, a new theory is gaining support that divides erectile dysfunction in complete, moderate, and minimal impotence on the basis of how much of the normal cavernosal smooth muscle architecture has been replaced by connective tissue. Assuming that young potent men have between 42 and 48% of cavernosal smooth muscle, completely impotent men have <30%, moderately impotent men have between 30 and 37%, and minimally impotent men have >39%.[44]

In addition, whereas NO is an important stimulus for vasodilation in the corpora, it is now recognized that the last step in producing relaxation of smooth muscle that allows more blood to be sequestered in the penis is the reduction of calcium ions within the smooth muscle. New drugs for impotence that facilitate calcium ion flux from the cell are under development. As research in this area advances, new mechanisms underlying potency and erectile dysfunction are being elucidated at a rapid rate. Stay tuned!

Are the Sexual Deficits of the 50s Essentially the Same in Both Sexes?

Estrogen deficiency from naturally occurring ovarian failure leads to decreased blood flow to the pelvis, eventually resulting in shrinkage of all external and internal sex organs. The clitoris, the homologue of the penis, for instance, loses its vascularity, is more heavily composed of fibrous tissue, and is less able to respond to external stimulation with a sustained tumescence. The vagina, a richly vascular elastic thick organ, is reduced to a few cell layers and its smooth muscles become more fibrotic and shrink, losing elasticity. The penis, which is hypoxic relative to other tissues, except in tumescence with sexual arousal or with REM sleep erectile enlargement, gradually loses its ability to respond to mental and manual stimulation, a state that is remarkably similar to the sexual problems of some postmenopausal problems. All of these observations would merely be interesting were it not for the explosion of research in how to prolong erectile capacity in men. The exciting implications of research in male erectile dysfunction are that the new findings in males are beginning to generate interest in exploring what may be done for women. The nonhormonal drugs that are being used for men with impotence are beginning to be thought of as a possible way to prevent or reverse some of women's sexual deficits. Could a phosphoesterase inhibitor that increases the concentration of cGMP in cavernosal tissues cause vasodilation in the penis and the clitoris? At this fresh point in pharmacological research, why not? For women in good health who want to take estrogens, such drugs then might be added to their regimen. For women who cannot or will not take estrogens, they may be used alone.

The Sexual Equilibrium in the 50s

These new gradual biological declines of both women and men affect each of the sexual function components—drive, motivation, wish, arousal, orgasm, and emotional satisfaction. What individuals bring to their partners, therefore, is different during this phase. As always in a sexual equilbrium, how their partners regard these new sexual characteristics will affect the frequency of sexual behavior and their emotional satisfaction from it. For a couple both aged 50, the wife may seem to be the limiting factor in their changed tenor of sexual behaviors. The husband's attitudes are crucial. Let 8 years pass, she may have long ago accommodated to her new sexual self but he is now the limiting factor in their again changing sexual equilibrium. It is her attitude that becomes crucial.

For some individuals of any age, these changes are too much. They are intensely frustrated by the new uncertainty of the outcome of their sexual behavior. Their private emotional responses to their diminishing but misunderstood sexual capacities create new obstacles. They begin to avoid attempting those activities that are painful, embarrassing, or unreliable. They say they are too tired. Physically healthy people in this decade are often tired earlier in the evening than before, but this is not the essence of the reason for sexual avoidance. Other individuals rise to the challenge, learn how to cope with the new diminishing sexual capacities, and keep the value of sexual behavior (see phase 3) firmly in view. They may even have sex earlier in the evenings, in the middle of the night, or use the mornings for this important behavior together. They do what they can comfortably do because their standards for what ought to be are no longer those of their 30s and 40s. They accept their declining capacities with sadness, but without partner derision. Orgasms occur. Reassuring touching occurs. Laughter can still break out during sex. Gratitude for the continuation of sexual activity—although nothing to rave about as in past years—may be felt and expressed to one another.

For men and women who are the regular sexual partners of individuals who are in a different physiological phase, there can be considerably more pressure and desperation to maintain potency. "I am fine now with my 38-year-old new wife, but what will happen in 2 or 3 years when I am in my early 60s?" "Will he lose sexual interest in me when I turn 50 like he did with his first wife?" Women who have noticed a distinct personal physiological decline and who are seeking partners may have developed a greater willingness to be sexually pleasing than they were earlier in their lives. Unattached men who have developed penile unreliability may begin to avoid social contact with women for the first time in many decades.

Clinicians often have a difficult time conceptualizing the sexual equilibrium in any age group. We prefer to think of sexual dysfunctions as related to the psychology or the physiology of the man or the woman. We have come to expect that the urologist will only dimly perceive the equilibrium, and primarily through the eyes of the man—the partner is either interested or not. We have also come to expect that the gynecologist will be more attentive to maintaining hormone-bathed pelvic structures than to the patient's interactions with her partner. If any professional can be expected to grasp the importance of the sexual equilibrium, it is the mental health professional. We are supposed to grasp the complexity of ordinary sexual interactions. Mental health professionals in the past have been as guilty of not conceptualizing the interactive effects of sexuality as the urologists and gynecologists. We used to focus on the intrapsychic or the intrapersonal aspects of sexual function and get waylaid by our ideological identifications. Hopefully, this is diminishing as we seek to understand more specific adult developmental problems. In this phase, it is as erroneous to assume that menopausal deficits are unimportant as it is to assume that men's sexual drives remain robust even if their penises do not.

All clinicians have vastly underestimated the effect of menopausal changes on women and their partners and most have similarly turned a blind eye to the loss of drive, sexual motivation, and erectile security of men in their late 50s. These are delicate painful matters, and patients often do not discuss them with their spouse, physician, or mental health professional. But if the clinician asks questions about sexual life in a manner that reflects knowledge about what is naturally occurring, all of this changes. Patients listen, learn, and become interested in what we have to offer psychologically, medically, and interpersonally to maintain their sexual lives together.

PHASE 5: FURTHER DECLINES IN OLDER AGE

The most useful predictor of sexual activity in people over age 60 is the success of their sexual adjustment in middle age. Those who have weathered the social and biological challenges of earlier phases still have an opportunity to have a sexual life with a partner. What we can expect, however, is that the aging effects that we began to observe in the 50s probably will continue. After age 60 it is far more difficult to separate the effects of healthy aging from those of illness, medication, and treatments for disease.

For example, the capacity to sequester blood in the penis and to maintain an erection seems to further diminish in the 60s. The percentage of men who acknowledge an inability to perform intercourse is approximately 60% at age 70. Male orgasmic attainment is more difficult. Many men after age 60 report that they sometimes cannot ejaculate. Although we like to tell the story of the 87-year-old man who was still having intercourse, and indeed there are some, they are a rarity. After age 60, the older heterosexual woman's sexual life depends on: having a man for a partner, his general health, his potency, her vaginal health, and her anticipation of sex as a pleasurable emotionally satisfying event.

To meet the challenge of maintaining a sexual life during healthy aging without medical intervention, the person has to make love with what one has. Hands and mouths are reliable, penises and vaginas are not. Artificial lubricants enable intercourse and the continuation of stimulation of the vulva for the woman's pleasure.

It is common for couples to end their sexual lives together because one or both members regard an erection as necessary to "get the job done" or regard nonintercourse sex as sick, immoral, or perverse. Such an ending also may end all affectionate behaviors in private because the man does not want to start something that he cannot finish and the woman, knowing how upset he is about his difficulty, does not initiate because she does not want him to feel badly. They may soothe themselves with the idea that they are too old for sex and all things come to an end.

Despite the cessation of activity in the sexual equilibrium, masturbation may continue both for men, with a less than full erection, and for women, with less than abundant lubrication, well into old age.

In the decades that are thought to represent early older age—60 to 79 years—the importance of separating the components of sexual desire into drive, motivation, and wish becomes clearer for clinicians. Many men and women still wish to behave sexually and those who have weathered the previous phases well do so. Sexual drive as recognized earlier in life from spontaneous urges for sex or lingering arousal from exciting stimuli in the environment do not have the same impact on people. Even explicit movies that people may have used in their 40s and 50s to augment their declining excitement may not yield the desired effect. Drive is diminished, yet in some couples and individuals behavior continues because they have mutual motives to behave sexually. Desire per se is not over, but the proportions of its components—drive, motive, and wish—change considerably in older ages.

PHASE 6: THE ARRIVAL OF ILLNESS

Serious, chronic, recurrent illnesses and their many treatments can occur at any stage of the life cycle. When they do, few individuals should expect to have their sexual components and sexual equilibrium unaffected. Few people at 60 have not had at least one episode of serious illness. Such illnesses occur more frequently as we age. The effects of breathlessness from chronic lung disease, medication for depression, impotence from prostatectomy, or radium scarring of the vagina that results from some uterine cancer therapy all change our sexual lives. Changes may occur because our sexual components are biologically altered, we regard ourselves differently now that our bodies are changed, or partners regard us differently. Regardless of the mechanism, the sex-

ual equilibrium shifts again. Although illness and its treatments are organic assaults on our sexual capacities, the organic assaults are often
temporary; the new views of ourselves and partners are not. Either organic or psychological assaults, if not thoughtfully managed, can end
our sexual lives at any age.

Breast cancer, for example, typically leads to some combination
of surgery, chemotherapy, radiation, and the use of tamoxifen, a
menopause-inducing estrogen blocker. These treatments physically
change the woman, her partner, and their sexual equilibrium. She usually survives her chemotherapy and radiation and eventually regains
her strength; her surgical area soon loses its soreness. She is not given
HRT because of the fear that estrogen will create tumor growth.
Tamoxifen-induced or -deepened menopause, with its attendant sexual
deficits, requires her to use external lubrication and come to grips with
the price that she has had to pay for the medical benefits of the drug.
Her reactions to these changes, her perception of her partner's reaction
to her bodily changes, his reaction to these changes, his perception of
her reactions to her new body—all are psychological consequences.

Prostate cancer often leads to total prostatectomy, which renders
many men unable to erect and some incontinent. Incontinence can create so much embarrassment that the man never gets the treatment for
impotence that is available. The woman may not mention sex again out
of kindness to her husband or because his incontinence prevents her
from thinking about sex with him. Sexual behavior and affection may
cease without any discussion.[45]

We should not forget that many illnesses affect men and women at
their so-called sexual prime. It is not generally polite to think of people
as relatively asexual but clinicians should not be surprised to learn that
their relatively young and reasonably coupled patients have little to no
satisfying sexual life. It is an accomplishment to manage life with a serious chronic illness and maintain a frequent satisfying sexual interaction. Clearly not impossible, but challenging.[46]

WHAT DETERMINES OUR SEXUAL FATE?

Our sexual fate is determined by many factors that derive from each
sexual phase. We hope that the challenges of couplehood—forming

and maintaining a sexual equilibrium of high quality, coping with multiple threats posed by disagreements, disappointments, illness and its treatment, gradual declines of the early aging processes—can be built on a good foundation of young adult sexual comfort. But even young adult sexual comfort cannot guarantee continued emotionally satisfying sexual expression with a partner; the couple must deal with their lives well. This includes understanding and effectively dealing with the challenges of phases 3 through 6. Willingness to discuss the subject together, to try new avenues of sexual expression, to maintain a sense of humor, and to keep some perspective about what has become of us as we age help a great deal.

REFERENCES

1. U.S. Congress, U.S. Office of Technology Assessment Vol. 3:1992.
2. Wise, P.M., Krajnak, K.M., and Kashon, M.L. Menopause: The aging of multiple pacemakers. *Science* 273:7–70, 1996.
3. Walling, M., Andersen, B.L., and Johnson, S.R. Hormonal replacement therapy for postmenopausal women: A review of sexual outcomes and related gynecologic effects. *Archives of Sexual Behavior* 19(2):119–137, 1990.
4. Sherwin, B.B. Sexuality and the menopause. In: G. Berg and M. Hammar (eds.), *The Modern Management of the Menopause.* Parthenon Publishing: New York, 1993, pp. 617–620.
5. Bachman, G.A. Influence of menopause on sexuality. *International Journal of Fertility and Menopausal Studies* (Suppl.) 40(1):16–22, 1995.
6. Greer, G. *The Change: Women, Aging, and the Menopause.* Knopf: New York, 1992.
7. Special Advisory Committee on Reproductive Physiology. *Menopause.* Minister of Supply and Services Canada, 1995.
8. Brambilla, D.K., and McKinlay, S.J. A prospective study of factors affecting age at menopause. *Journal of Clinical Epidemiology* 42(11):1031–1039, 1989.
9. McCoy, N.L. The menopause and sexuality. In: R. Sitruk-Ware and W.H. Utian (eds.), *The Menopause and Hormone Replacement Therapy:Facts and Controversies.* Dekker: New York, 1991, pp. 73–100.
10. Longcope, C. The endocrinology of the menopause. In: R.A. Lobo (ed.), *Treatment of Menopausal Women: Basic and Clinical Aspects.* Raven Press: New York, 1994, pp. 47–56.
11. Longcope, C., Jaffe, W., and Griffing, G. Production rates of androgens and oestrogens in post-menopausal women. *Maturitas* 3(3–4):215–223, 1981.
12. Masters, W.H., and Johnson, V. *Human Sexual Response.* Little, Brown: Boston, 1966.
13. Bretschneider, J.G., and McCoy, N.L. Sexual behavior and interest in healthy 80- to 102-year olds. *Archives of Sexual Behavior* 17:109–129, 1988.
14. McCoy, N.L. Survey research on the menopause and women's sexuality. In: G. Berg and M. Hammar (eds.), *The Modern Management of the Menopause.* Parthenon Publishing: New York, 1993, pp. 581–588.
15. Hallström, T. Sexuality of women in middle age: The Gotteborg Study. *Journal of Biosocial Science* (Suppl.) 6:165–175, 1979.

16. McCoy, N.L., and Davidson, J.M. A longitudinal study of the effects of menopause on sexuality. *Maturitas* 7:203–210, 1985.

17. American Society for Reproductive Medicine. *Menopause* (Patient Information Series). Birmingham, 1996.

18. American College of Obstetrics and Gynecology Patient Education. *The Menopause Years.* December, 1995.

19. Nathorst-Böös, J., Wiklund, I., Mattsson, L.A., Sandin, K., and von Schouitz, B. Is sexual life influenced by transdermal estrogen therapy? A double blind placebo controlled study in postmenopausal women. *Acta Obstetricia et Gynecologia Scandinavica* 72:656–660, 1993.

20. Studd, J. Continuation rates with cyclical and continuous regimes of oral estrogens and progestogens (editorial). *Menopause* 3(4):181–182, 1966.

21. Longcope, C. Adrenal and gonadal steroid secretion in normal females. *Journal of Clinical Endocrinology and Metabolism* 15:215–228, 1986.

22. Sherwin, B.B. A comparative analysis of the role of androgen in human male and female sexual behavior: Behavioral specificity, critical thresholds, and sensitivity. *Psychobiology* 16: 416–425, 1988.

23. Sherwin, B.B., Gelfand, M.M., and Brender, W. Androgen enhances motivation in females: A prospective, cross-over study of sex steroid administration in the surgical menopause. *Psychosomatic Medicine* 47: 339–351, 1985.

24. Rako, S. *The Hormone of Desire: The Truth about Sexuality, Menopause, and Testosterone.* Harmony Books: New York, 1996.

25. Plouffe, L., and Cohen, D. The role of androgens in menopausal hormone replacement therapy. In: J. Lorrain (ed.), *Comprehensive Management of Menopause*. Springer-Verlag: Berlin, 1994, pp. 397–408.

26. Dopay, B., Balos, R., and Willard, N. Improved menopausal symptom relief with estrogen–androgen therapy. Poster-16. *Abstracts: Seventh Annual Meeting of North American Menopause Society in Menopause* 3(4):233, 1996.

27. Sarrel, P.M. Laser Doppler measurement of peripheral blood flow. In: M. Notelovitz and P.A. van Keep (eds.), *The Climacteric in Perspective*. MTP Press: Lancaster, 1986, pp. 161–175.

28. Semmens, J.P., Tsai, C.C., Semmens, E.C., and Loadholt, C.B. Effects of estrogen therapy on vaginal physiology during menopause. *Obstetrics Gynecology* 66:15–18, 1985.

29. Special Advisory Committee on Reproductive Physiology to the Drugs Directorate Health Protection Branch Health Canada. *Menopause*. Minister of National Health and Welfare, Canada, 1995, p. 43.

30. McCoy, N.L. Sexual issues for postmenopausal women. *Topics in Geriatric Rehabilitation* 12(4):1–12, 1997.

31. Cawood, E.H.H., and Bancroft, J. Steroid hormones, the menopause, sexuality, and well-being of women. *Psychological Medicine* 26:925–936, 1996.

32. Leiblum, S., Bachmann, G., Kenmann, E., Colburn, D., and Swartzman, L. Vaginal atrophy in the postmenopausal woman: The importance of sexual activity and hormones. *JAMA* 249:2195–2198, 1983.

33. Cutler, W.B., Garcia, C.R., and McCoy, N. Perimenopausal sexuality. *Archives of Sexual Behavior* 16(3):225–234, 1987.

34. Ettinger, B., Li, D.K., and Klein, R. Continuation of postmenopausal hormone replacement therapy: Comparison of cyclic versus continuous combined schedules. *Menopause* 3(4):185–189, 1966.

35. Isaacs, A.J., Britton, A.R., and McPherson, K. Utilisation of hormone replacement by women doctors. *British Medical Journal* 311:1399–1401, 1995.

36. Schiavi, R.C., Schreiner-Engel, P., Mandeli, J., Schanzer, H., Cohen, E. Healthy aging and male sexual function. *American Journal of Psychiatry* 147(6):766–771, 1990.
37. Feldman, H.A., Goldstein, I., Hatzichristou, D.G., Krane, R.J., and McKinlay, J.B. Impotence and its medical and psychological correlates: Results of the Massachusetts male aging study. *Journal of Urology* 151:54–61, 1994.
38. Mulhall, J.P., and Goldstein, I. Epidemiology of erectile dysfunction. In: J.J. Mulcahy (ed.), *Diagnosis and Management of Male Sexual Dysfunction.* Igaku-Shoin: New York, 1996, pp. 1–11.
39. Laumann, E.O. *Sex in America.* University of Chicago Press: Chicago, 1995.
40. Love, S. Sometimes mother nature knows best. Op-Ed. *New York Times* March 20, 1997, p. A19.
41. Wespes, E., deGoes, P.M., and Schulman, C. Vascular impotence: Focal or diffuse penile disease. *Journal of Urology* 1435–1436, 1992.
42. Althof, S.E., and Seftel, A.D. The evaluation and management of erectile dysfunction in clinical sexuality. *Psychiatric Clinics of North America* 18(1):171–192, 1995.
43. Broderick, G.A. Noninvasive arterial investigation of the patient complaining of erectile dysfunction using the color duplex Doppler ultrasound. In: J.J. Mulcahy (ed.), *Diagnosis and Management of Male Sexual Dysfunction.* Igaku-Shoin: New York, 1996, pp.111–112.
44. Goldstein, I. Pharmacologic treatment of male sexual dysfunction: New frontiers and challenges. Lecture presented at Society for Sex Therapy and Research Meeting in Chicago, March 1997.
45. Fagan, P.J., and Blum, L.H. Issues in the psychotherapeutic therapy of of sexual dysfunction following radical retropubic prostatectomy. In: R.C. Rosen and S.R. Leiblum (eds.), *Case Studies in Sex Therapy.* Guilford Press: New York, 1995, pp. 193–208.
46. Curry, S., and Levine, S.B., The impact of Systemic Lupus Erythematosis on women's sexual functioning. *J. Rheumatology* 21(12): 2254–2260, 1994.

Extramarital Sexual Affairs in Mid-Life I: Meaning-Making

Madness need not be all breakdown. It may also be breakthrough.
It is potential liberation and renewal as well as enslavement and
existential death.
—Rudyard Kipling[1]

SEXUAL ACTING OUT

What Shall We Call Them?

The four types of extramarital sexual liaisons that are mentioned in this chapter share one vital characteristic: Their intent is to be secret from a committed partner. Beyond this, surreptitious unions seem to vary considerably in purpose, duration, and impact.

1. *Affair.* As used in this chapter, this term implies an evolving personal attachment between two clandestine lovers. The actual affair usually begins at some emotional point of psychological intimacy before sexual consummation, although the parties may only acknowledge their bond after sexual activity together. Consummation not only deepens the bond but also gives birth to a set of unverbalized expectations for future talking, sharing time together, and sexual interaction. An affair involves intimate psychological knowledge of the other person, which along with the sexual implies some degree of internal

bond to the lover. The end of an affair typically is at least privately painful.

2. *Just-sex.* Many surreptitious liaisons are sexual, quickly so, but carry no emotional, social, or sexual obligation beyond the original physical acts. These are "just-sex." Liaisons with prostitutes, pickups at bars or parties, convention flings, or other one-night stands are heterosexual examples. Arrangements made at parks, bookstores, or bathhouses are male homosexual examples. The sexual acting out of just-sex, because it involves no intimate psychological knowledge of the sexual partner does not generate an attachment bond. There generally is no pain of separation or loss when just-sex arrangements are over.

3. *Making-do sex.* I know of no good single term to describe the abortive relationships that are neither an affair nor just-sex. Sometimes described as casual or convenient sex, these relaxed-sounding terms belie the fact that the behavior is the product of varying degrees of deception of the new partner and gross ambivalence—filled with fits and starts, confusions, advantage-taking, and wavering. After a while, both partners come to realize that their future as a couple is quite limited; they were just making-do. The pain over termination of the relationship is primarily guilt or embarrassment; these endings, however, are primarily relief.

4. *Imaginary partner sex.* Until recently, this category was largely a male form of extramarital sex that was of interest to clinicians because of its association with partner avoidance and intense dependence on masturbation. Explicit still pictures, videotapes, or strip shows have traditionally captivated heterosexual men's erotic imagination in this problematic way. Homosexual male counterparts have included explicit male-on-male videos and opportunities for voyeuristic excitement at movies, bathhouses, and parks. But now, clinicians are seeing men and women who discover imaginary sex while talking to strangers on the phone or via conversations on the internet. This is quasi-imaginary quasi-extramarital sex. People can become quite attached to these forms of sexual behaviors, and, paradoxically, they may be the most difficult to give

up. Many people describe their ongoing need for these forms of sexual behavior, and their failed attempts to stop the use of these props as "addiction."

Acting Out

Mental health professionals often indiscriminantly refer to any of these four forms of extramarital sex as acting out. Our clinical responses are often to delineate the intrapsychic or interpersonal dilemmas whose affects are being indirectly expressed through these sexual behaviors. Acting out is often assumed to be a manifestation of either individual or couple's psychopathology. This is sometimes a justifiable assumption. The evidence that sexual acting out can be a form of psychopathology comes from several sources:

- Acting out can be self-destructively dangerous. The secret forbidden nature of the activity can readily become preoccupying or "addicting." Even an affair with a real person can feel addicting.
- Considerable emotional distress appears in the couple when any of these activities is discovered by partners. When a partner's affair is not just another problem caused by an obvious longstanding psychopathology, the discovery of an affair usually has a dramatic capacity to generate suffering.
- Some extramarital sexual behaviors are strongly associated with major psychiatric illnesses, character disorders, or paraphilia.[2] Disorders such as hypomania, cocaine abuse, psychopathic personality, and exhibitionism strain the person's capacity to remain faithful to the spouse and strain the spouse's capacity for patience and commitment.
- There is a long psychodynamic tradition of explaining extramarital sexual behaviors in terms of developmental psychopathology, particularly of preoedipal and oedipal varieties.[3]

Although I agree that much extramarital sex may helpfully be viewed as a manifestation of a maladaptive mental state, this chapter emphasizes an understanding of the more immediate genesis and consequences of mid-life affairs, that is, extramarital acting out from the first category. For many of these individuals the question is not simply one of psychopathology; it is more existential—"To be faithful or to be unfaithful."

An Incomplete Registry of Extramarital Situations

Consider this seemingly redundant long list:

1. A man has an affair.
2. A woman has an affair.
3. An engaged person has an affair.
4. A person has an affair soon after marriage, in the early phases of evolving a new sexual equilibrium.
5. A person in a long-established relationship has an affair.
6. A man has an affair when his spouse is showing physiological decline in the perimenopausal–menopausal era.
7. A woman has an affair when her spouse is showing physiological decline in his 50s.
8. A person has an affair after several years of the partner's unexplained, unexplored unwillingness to have sex.
9. A person has an affair after years of an unsatisfying relationship lacking in psychological intimacy.
10. A man has an affair when his spouse is chronically seriously physically ill.
11. A woman has an affair when her spouse is chronically seriously physically ill.
12. A person has an affair when the spouse is chronically seriously mentally ill.
13. A single or divorced woman has an affair with a married man.
14. A single or divorced man has an affair with a married woman.
15. Two young married people have an affair.
16. Two middle-aged married people have an affair.
17. Two older married people have an affair.
18. A married man has a homosexual affair.
19. A married man has homosexual just-sex with a stranger.
20. A married man has sex with a male prostitute.
21. A married woman has a lesbian affair.

22. A married man has sex with a female prostitute.
23. A married man has just-sex with a woman, a stranger, while out of town.
24. A married man has imaginary masturbatory sex with a woman, a stranger, on the Internet.
25. A married woman has just-sex with a man, a stranger, while out of town.
26. A married woman has imaginary masturbatory sex with a man, a stranger, on a phone call arranged by a company whose business is bringing people together for sexual chats.
27. A making-do relationship is developed during a couple's long vocational geographic separation.
28. A man in a committed gay relationship has an affair with a man.
29. A man in a committed gay relationship has just-sex with another man.
30. A man in a committed gay relationship has an affair with a woman.
31. A lesbian in a committed relationship has a homosexual affair.
32. A lesbian in a committed relationship has an affair with a man.
33. A person in the armed forces is stationed away from his or her spouse in a foreign land where significant danger exists and begins a just-sex arrangement with someone in the same situation.
34. A woman who always has lived on the verge of poverty, discovers that her man has been with another woman.
35. A woman of considerable independent financial means discovers her husband's infidelity.
36. A priest, committed to celibacy, has homosexual just-sex with a stranger.
37. A priest, committed to celibacy, has a longstanding homosexual affair.
38. A priest, committed to celibacy, has a heterosexual affair.
39. A clergyman whose religion does not require celibacy falls in love and has an affair with a congregant.
40. A married faithful 45-year-old man says he is addicted to heterosexual pornography and imagines controlling, dominating, and humiliating his attractive 20-year-old female partners.

41. An unhappily married woman with children has periodic brief sexual liaisons that she abruptly ends.
42. A person has a second affair during marriage.
43. A middle-aged psychotherapist has his fifth sexual relationship with a patient during the psychotherapy sessions.
44. A middle-aged psychotherapist has her first sexual relationship with a patient, but ends the relationship first.

Meaning-Makers

To emphasize the fact that the meanings of affairs vary with each individual involved, I sometimes refer to people as *meaning-makers*. In the typical previously clandestine affair that comes to psychiatric attention, the usual cast of meaning-makers includes: the person having the affair, the person with whom the affair is conducted, the committed partner, the mental health professional, and possibly a confidant of one of the lovers. Therapists become immersed in the meanings of those who consult them. In conjoint therapy with a couple attempting to recover from the aftermath of an affair, it is readily apparent, for example, that each involved person, even the person not in the room, attributes distinctly different meanings to the affair. The clinician's role is often to order these meanings in an understandable and useful fashion.

Unanswered Questions from the Registry

The long list of extramarital situations suggests a number of questions. Do men and women tend to experience and view affairs differently? Do affairs evoke differing meanings in different parts of the life cycle? Are just-sex experiences significantly easier for the committed partner to bear than affairs? Are just-sex experiences less guilt provoking for the unfaithful person? Do gay men and lesbians have less expectation for partner fidelity than their heterosexual counterparts? Does lower expectation for fidelity for any reason (such as a long history of economic disadvantage) affect how infidelity is experienced? Does the meaning of an affair stem from a grasp of what the negative consequences may be? Are religious vows of celibacy comparable to marriage in terms of meanings of partner sexual experiences? Is extramarital sex in cyberspace less disruptive than physical contact sex? Is extramarital sex that occurs with a current or former therapist more dangerous than affairs in general? I suspect that the answer to each of these questions is likely to be "yes," but my impressions are not based on clinical science, just personal observation.

HOW AFFAIRS BEGIN

Flirting

Flirtation is early courtship behavior, a means of getting the erotic attention of another. It often occurs in public settings, disguised as ordinary politeness. Its observable mechanisms involve prolonged eye contact, apparent interest or enjoyment in the person's conversation, standing or sitting close to the person, and a slight excess of innocuous touching. No verbal expressions of personal interest are necessary to create the excitement that comes from the realization that he or she is "interested in me."

Sometimes, flirtation is offered so subtly that no one, including the person it is intended to interest, perceives it. Sometimes, it is sufficiently subtle that only the intended recognizes it. Some flirting, however, is so obvious that many in the room know that it is occurring. Such flirting strikes many as outrageous. It is not generally considered to be a compliment to be called a flirt. In fact, some flirts are perceived to be socially dangerous.

Flirtation is portrayed by many of its practitioners as a harmless social game.[4] It may be that, and it may be much more. For the flirting person, the behavior creates a tantalizing, promising, exciting uncertainty. People flirt for many reasons:

- To make social occasions less boring
- To affirm one's attractiveness, social worth, or power to provoke interest in others
- To seek a sexual liaison
- To pretend to themselves that they have more relationship possibilities than they know that they have
- To celebrate the overcoming of one's former social shyness and sense of social inadequacy

- To provoke sexual desire in oneself or another person
- To present a false impression to others of oneself as a comfortable sexual person

Flirting per se does not generally earn the disparaging label of "a flirt." Flirtation may be occasionally initiated in response to attractions to another, fantasies about a more exciting sex or interpersonal life, consumption of alcohol, and the need to find a distraction from some nonsexual frustration.

When the Flirtation Is Over

The flirtation signal is sometimes received with serious interest. Intimate talk, setting up the next occasion for more psychologically intimate talk, and escalation of intrapsychic arousal and erotic imagery can then quickly occur. The harmless social game takes on a new seriousness. Flirtation is then over. The contingency that was being played with has been transformed into a new reality. Men and women who have decided that these liaisons are part of the pleasure of living their lives can perfect the process of spotting, alerting, and negotiating with another to an impressive degree.

The Mid-Life Marital Paradox as Background for an Affair

By mid-life many individuals have already been numbed by their conclusion that they are not sufficiently satisfied in their marital relationship. They may be disappointed about what does or does not happen within the home, bedroom, or social activities. Or they may reach their conclusions from the frequency and strength of their fantasies or behaviors with others. However they arrive at their judgment, they may find themselves preoccupied with their perception that their love for their partner is moribund or has already died. Or, "Did I ever really love this person?"

What they know with certainty is that they desire something fresher, more exciting. They want something less encumbered by their appraisal of their partner, less burdened by their partner's appraisal of them. They imagine beginning anew but, of course, the reality of their commitment immovably stands there like a fortress. A defense arises: They pretend that they are not seriously entrapped within a marriage and family or within a culturally sanctioned commitment—they flirt a little.

A friend may have recently decided to divorce or take a lover, but such a drastic step may not feel like a realistic possibility for the person we are considering here. A search for safer interests may begin—in work, recreation, children, or the community. An otherwise unexplained period of depression, however, may appear. Because the person may not be willing to acknowledge to him- or herself this state of feeling unhappily married, a clinician may consider this to reflect a diminution of cerebral or limbic synaptic serotonin. The mood of depression with its many classical symptoms may be summarized by perceiving it as a reaction to the prediction of the future, "Is this what my life is to be?"

Some feel rebellious against what fate has brought to them. The possibility of beginning anew, of revitalizing oneself in a new relationship, of behaving differently with someone else keeps appearing in consciousness. The internal voice whispers repeatedly "Have an affair!" Its pleasures are deliciously imagined; its dangers are minimized.

"But what will happen to my partner and children if the affair is discovered?" "Can the honest me tolerate the tantalizing dishonesty?" "Didn't I always want to be faithful?" These thoughts may be dominated by others such as: "Oh stop being so self-depriving! Others do it, it isn't the end of the world! Its just a little dalliance, an experience. What if my partner has been doing it and I foolishly don't have any awareness of it? Just make the ground rules clear from the beginning. I'll look for somebody who is looking for something that fits with what I am looking for. So I will no longer think of myself as honest a person as I used to be. Since when is honesty an absolute thing?"

Most of these internal mental events are merely private dramas that go nowhere. But, affairs do occur. The unwary spouse angers the person, a vocational success or failure occurs, another person flirts, a high school or college reunion occurs, a new co-worker is hired, a distraction is needed from the pain of a looming death of a family member—something occurs, and it begins. Whatever the final provocation, the person decides, actively makes a choice to participate at every step along the way.

Conceptualizing the Paradox

The paradox that forces itself on the middle-aged person is between oneself as socially committed and mentally uncommitted, between honesty and deception, between what one wants to do to revitalize oneself and how secret one wants to keep this motive. Many theorists have emphasized the tolerance of paradox that occurs during mid-life. They have not emphasized, however, that some individuals cannot tolerate the paradox without having an affair. The less mature act out the paradox; they live it rather than simply feel and know about it. During the middle years, in contrast to the young adult years, it is harder to imagine that the person does not know that he or she has made a decision. An irresistable force overcoming reason, or being overwhelmed by sexual attraction may be an understandable defense for a young adult, but it is harder to use as a psychological explanation as one accumulates more life experience. Middle-aged self-awareness is now far more complex. Black and white have become gray zones, potential has become a word largely applied to younger people, and the end of life opportunities has taken on a new emotional valence. Mature middle-aged people also have affairs but they realize that they have chosen to do so. The affair then tranforms the person from a mere intellectual grasp of the contradictions of existence to an intense emotional grasp of living with paradox.

THE CLINICIAN'S PERSPECTIVES

The Therapist's Gender

The gender of the therapist may be vital in creating clinical experience. Most of the betrayed people I have an opportunity to see are women (3:1). Most of the people initiating affairs, having just-sex, making-do, or having imaginary partner sex are men. My female colleagues also have much experience with betrayed women but a larger percentage of their practices consist of women discussing their extramarital relationships. Select female colleagues hear a lot more about the sexual liaisons of lesbians in committed relationships.

The Mind of the Betrayed

It is not unusual for a clinician to be consulted when a person discovers that the partner is having an affair. We then have an opportunity to observe the thoughts, feelings, defenses, modifying circumstances, and coping strategies of the betrayed.

In the midst of their crises, three matters confuse the betrayed:

1. the intensity of their emotions
2. the expected time course of their feelings ("How long will I feel this way?")
3. the uncertain answers to a surprisingly large number of recurring questions, many of which arise at the same time

The Questions of the Betrayed

The betrayed of either sex or orientation often struggle with some or most of the following matters:

1. Why did this happen?
2. Does this mean that something is wrong with me physically, sexually, interpersonally, or psychologically?
3. Does this mean that something is wrong with our relationship?
4. Does this mean that something is wrong with my partner?
5. Is this just the way most people of that sex or orientation are?
6. Why do I feel this array of emotions: sadness, anxiety, anger, guilt, embarrassment, desperation, sexual desire for my partner, aversion for my partner, love, vengefulness?
7. Should I tell anyone about this? My friends, my parents, our children?
8. What else do I not know about my partner's behaviors?
9. Will I, does anyone, ever get over this?
10. Will I ever be able to forgive my partner?
11. Will I ever be able to forget this?
12. Will I be able to trust my partner again?
13. Will I be able to trust any partner again?
14. How can I make my partner realize what I am going through?
15. How do I best manage this? What will be the consequences of:
    • Seeking counseling?

- Consulting a divorce attorney?
- Having a retaliatory affair?
- Refusing to do anything for my partner for a while?
- Reading some books about affairs?
- Pretending that I intend to leave?
- Letting this quietly blow over?

16. Shall I think of myself as a fool?
17. Shall I take this opportunity to end this relationship?
18. Does it now matter to me that I previously had an extramarital experience?

The Coping Styles of the Betrayed

Clinicians can readily recognize a range of coping styles among the betrayed. At one pole are those patient, understanding responses, heavy with personal responsibility, and organized by the quick self-knowledge of "I want my partner back!" At the other extreme are the responses of indignant vengeful outrage, seeking immediate aggressive action, and organized by the decision that "My partner is history!" Most initial responses fall between these extremes.

The Therapist's Role

What the clinician has to say to the betrayed person depends a great deal on the coping styles being used at the moment. Therapists should pay attention to their patients' emotions and help them to succinctly express them. Therapists can helpfully distinguish those feelings that are likely to last a long time and those that are more transient. The emotions are tied to the questions; paying attention to either the emotion or the question helps with both. Therapists should generally understand that, although the questions are good ones, they do not actually know the answers to many of them. As long as one listens well with interest and appreciation of the pain and uncertainty, the betrayed seem to find relief in sharing their experience.

Clinicians may wonder what factors influence a middle-aged person's reactions to an affair. Matters such as where people are in their personal maturation, their private personal commitment to their partner, their value system, their children, their financial situation, whether it is a first or repeated affair experience, seem relevant. There are five reasons why we should be careful about such speculations, however: (1) Reactions proceed over time as the person digests what the threat is and how he or she feels about it; (2) the influence of the modifying factors may be small compared to the power of the betrayal alone; (3) after an affair, the relationship may be repaired in many important ways, yet remain forever changed by the experience of betrayal; (4) mental health professionals have never been much good at predicting; (5) most importantly, the meanings of meaning-makers are highly idiosyncratic.

The Therapist Experiencing the Betrayed

Clinicians cannot sit through too many betrayed people's experiences without realizing what they do not know about the subject. The questions that often occur to me and how I impressionistically answer them follow:

- Have affairs been systematically studied? (To an impressive degree, they have not been. The methodological challenges are great. How many people will even admit to their affair? When affairs have been studied, the effects seem to be strongly negative in terms of divorce and marital devitalization.[5])
- Have I missed helping people in the past because I failed to realize that the origin of anxiety and depressive symptoms was the discovery of infidelity? (Probably.)
- Can affairs have an ameliorative impact on the individual or couple with or without my assistance? (Yes, particularly if the aggrieved person can stop recalling his or her memories with anxiety, rage, jealousy, and paranoia. This is often where the therapist comes in.[6])
- Can I work with the couple if I know more about the person's present and past affairs than the betrayed does? (This is a very difficult challenge that seems to frequently limit the quality of the therapeutic relationship.)
- Was the infidelity "the result" of poor judgment caused by a readily apparent psychiatric illness? (Sometimes, but the deeper issue may still be the appraisal of the unfaithful person's

character; the psychiatric illness may be a minor or major miti-
gating factor. Clinicians should be careful that they do not consider that one of these illnesses is ***the*** cause of the affair. We can
provide the facts to our patient—for instance, manic patients
have traditionally been described as having poor social judgment and reduced inhibitions and become involved sexually
outside of their committed relationships. It is the betrayed person's decision how much emphasis to place on diagnosable psychiatric illness.)

- Was the affair a manifestation of another conspicuous or problematic character trait such as self-centeredness, insensitivity,
  grandiosity, entitlement, passive-aggressiveness, or impulsiv-
  ity? (The therapist and the betrayed person may profitably
  struggle with this issue together without it detracting from the
  unfaithful person's responsibility for the original decision.)
- Has this person's behavior created a problematic situation that
  the partner dealt with by behaving sexually outside the relationship? (The therapist and the betrayed person may profitably
  struggle with this issue together, but not too soon.)
- How do I now feel about affairs? (Do not kid yourself, you have
  attitudes!)

  - Could I ever do this to my partner? (Probably "yes," under
    some circumstances.)
  - Does my past—no affair, one affair, several affairs—influ-
    ence how I view this person's dilemmas? (Don't assume that
    you can be completely objective.)
  - Is my countertransference—moral outrage, guilty anxiety in
    the patient's presence, or my need for the patient to be proac-
    tive—interfering with my work with this person? (Be alert!)

The early experiences with the betrayed can be quite emotionally
evocative. Most experienced clinicians can recall their first opportunities to work with the betrayed. The most shocking experience that I
have had was with a woman brought to me by her sheepish husband in
mid-July. Their initial presentation led to me assume for 30 minutes
that she had discovered his affair "over Memorial Day weekend." It
turned out that the discovery occurred 7 years ago! Such extreme reactions are quite sad, frightening, and thankfully rare. But even more

ordinary reactions continue for a long time. And they may continue subjectively many years after the partner thinks that the person is over it. Working with the betrayed can be difficult, but probably is best balanced over time by opportunities to participate in the mental life of those who have betrayed.

The Mind of the Person Having the Affair

It can be quite difficult to tell a therapist about an affair. Perhaps because of shame or because we are being interviewed to ascertain our attitudes, several sessions can go by without being told about the liaison. I have conducted marital and individual therapies only to discover later, sometimes quite a bit later, that a spouse (of either sex) had been having an affair during therapy. Even when people speak at their first session about having an affair, telling *all* about it usually is quite onerous. Three aspects are particularly difficult: (1) the knowledge of why they participated, (2) the direct and indirect promises made to the new partner (including personal hopes for an improved life), and (3) the lies told to the new partner.

Nonetheless, we learn from what people tell us and how they reveal it. These men and women teach us about the familiar thoughts, feelings, defenses, modifying circumstances, and coping strategies used by the person involved in an affair.

It is not generally useful to search for the *type of individual* who has an affair. U.S. data from different eras—1940s to 1970—created the impression that approximately 50% of married men and about 20% of married women admitted to at least one extramarital experience. Divorced women have about 2.5 times the likelihood of having had an extramarital experience than currently married women.[7] Such data cannot be given a great deal of credence because of methodological difficulties, the tendency not to reveal such information, and the numerous factors that modify prevalence figures. Earlier estimates range widely from study to study—for instance, 26 to 55% for men and 21 to 45% for women. In a more recent survey done as part of the HIV risk, individuals between ages 18 and 75 were asked by phone about their sex partners in the last 12 months.[8] Men were more likely than women to have had extramarital sex—2.9 versus 1.5%. All studies have displayed the greater tendency of men to have extramarital vaginal intercourse—whether measured by within the last year or ever—but recent studies of younger women suggest that the differences are diminishing. For African Americans and Hispanics but not Caucasians, church attendance was associated with lower extramarital sex rates. After considering many studies, Brown, a clinician, estimated that 70% of marriages experience an affair.[9] Two recent methodologically careful surveys have suggested that 24.5[10] and 22.7%[11] of men and 15 and 11.6% of women have ever had vaginal intercourse with someone other than their spouse while married. Although the validity of all studies remain uncertain, some data suggest that today's married women have affairs about 10 years earlier than the previous generation.[12] Women's extramarital activity tends to increase between ages 30 and 50 and then decrease, whereas men's activity tends to be consistent until the 60s.[11] The survey researcher's view of the phenomenon of extramarital sex is different from the clinician's not only in scientific care and acceptability, but also in what can be learned about the activity. Clinicians need information from the social scientists to help them not lose perspective. The clinician's perspective is a close-in one, filled with powerful emotion and meaning, and plagued by the lack of sociological perspective.

Two phenomena are common among those who seek help after initiating an affair: (1) In answer to many of the therapist's questions, the reply comes, "I did not think about that." (2) During the discussion of the current complex situation, the person sighs deeply and remarks, "If I only would have known what this would bring." This is not to say that people invariably regret their affairs; some in fact cherish them and feel that the affairs were worth the problems that ensued. Nonetheless, they want to discuss them because so much is cognitively and affectively swirling within them.

Here are some of the issues that seem to be inherent in the experience of having an evolving relationship with a person outside of the marriage:

1. Am I doing this because my partner is so unsatisfying?
2. Am I doing this because I have lost respect for my partner?
3. Am I doing this because I am angry, deeply resentful, of my partner?
4. Am I doing this because I want to have this, I deserve to have this, I need this?

5. Am I doing this because of serendipity, a chance I decided to take advantage of?
6. Am I doing this because it would be too ugly to stop it?
7. How am I to think of myself now? I have become such a liar, yet I am generally an honest person.
8. Do I really want to stop this relationship?
9. If I devise a plan to stop, will I implement it?
10. Whom shall I hurt? Whether I stay, leave, or continue the affair, I will be deeply hurting somebody.
11. What am I to do now? Even if I implement the best plan I can think of, people, including me, will still be hurt.
12. If I return to my partner, will I be trusted?
13. If I stay with my lover, will I be trusted?
14. Why do I feel such an array of my emotions about my spouse: anger, guilt, pleased, embarrassed, nervous, irritated, disappointed, and afraid?
15. Does the grief that I feel when I decide or try to end the relationship mean that I love the person?
16. How can I tell the difference between loving and enjoying this person?
17. Would I be better off leaving my marriage?
18. Should I stay married just for my children?
19. What will my future be with my children if I leave their other parent?
20. What will be the future of my children if I leave?
21. I am a mess when I think about my betraying my partner. Should I try not to think about it?
22. I am just looking for love, another improved variety relationship, I just want to be a happy person. Am I kidding myself that I could be happy?
23. Who might be of help to me? A friend, a clergy, my physician, a therapist?
24. Are there any good books on the subject of having affairs?
25. Am I crazy?

Clinicians often see men and women after they have been discovered or after their affair has generated intense guilt, sexual dysfunction, or marital deterioration. But on occasion, a thoughtful person not in crisis finds the complexity of his or her life reason to consult a clinician. We then discuss these issues in detail over time, the patient weighs them in importance, and some decision is eventually made. This is, of course, exactly what the clinician attempts to do with those whose distress is more acute.

A Vignette

A 43-year-old politician originally sought help with his wife because of his continuing indecision about whether to leave the family for his never-married lover of 3 years. Everyone in the system—wife, three teenage daughters, lover, and he—had become highly symptomatic. For the last year, he had left each woman twice with the announcement of having made a final decision. Each time, however, he missed the other too much. He was living on the cellular phone secretly calling the other one. Although "not serious," he was beginning to think that the only way out was suicide. This vignette is from the tenth visit. Only he and I are present, his wife having previously decided that he needed me more than she did and that if anyone could save their marriage it would be me. At this visit I told him about Anthony Storr's book, *Solitude*.[13] I suggested that he go off by himself for a week and think this out, weighing his desires against the costs to himself and his family and friends about which we had previously discussed.

> *I call what you have a dilemma. Many problems have elegant solutions but a dilemma is a problem without a painless solution. Make no mistake— your dilemma is an unenviably terrible one: Whatever you decide, it will be quite difficult for a long time. But it is time for a real decision. Please remember that whatever you decide, you will have to work everyday to make it a good decision. You may not end up with either woman or a family. Go decide!*

So he did. He chose his lover because of his sense of the promise of a greater emotional and physical love than he was experiencing with his wife.

REFERENCES

1. Kipling, R. *Plain Tales from the Hills*. 'On the Strength of a Likeness' Excerpted from *Compton's Reference Collection 1996*. Copyright (c) 1995 Compton's NewMedia, 1995.

2. Levine, S.B. The paraphilias. In: B. Sadock and H.I. Kaplan (eds.), *Comprehensive Textbook of Psychiatry*. Williams & Wilkins: Baltimore, in press.

3. Kernberg, O. *Love Relations: Normality and Pathology*. Yale University Press: New Haven, 1995.

4. Phillips, A. On flirtation: Psychoanalytic essays on the uncommitted life. *On Flirtation: An Introduction*. Harvard University Press: Cambridge, MA, 1994, pp. xvii–xxv.

5. Charney, I.W., and Parnass, S. The impact of extramarital relationships on the continuation of marriages. *Journal of Sex and Marital Therapy* 21(2):100–115, 1995.

6. Scharff, D.E. Truth and consequence in sex and marital therapy: The revelation of secrets in the therapeutic setting. *Journal of Sex and Marital Therapy* 4:35–49, 1978.

7. Hunt, M. *Sexual Behavior in the 1970s*. Dell Publishing: New York, 1974.

8. Choi, K., Catania, J.A., and Dolcini, M.M. Extramarital sex and HIV risk behavior among US adults: Results from the National AIDS Behavioral Survey. *American Journal of Public Health* 84(12):2003–2007, 1994.

9. Brown, E. *Patterns of Infidelity and Their Treatment*. Brunner/Mazel: New York, 1992.

10. Laumann, E.O., Gagnon, J.H., Michael, R.T., and Michaels, S. *The Social Organization of Sexuality: Sexual Practices in the United States*. University of Chicago Press: Chicago, 1994.

11. Weiderman, M.W. Extramarital sex: Prevalence and correlates in a national survey. *The Journal of Sex Research* 34(2):167–174, 1997.

12. Lawson, A. *Adultery: An Analysis of Love and Betrayal*. Basic Books: New York, 1988.

13. Storr, A. *Solitude: A Return to the Self*. Free Press: New York, 1988.

Extramarital Sexual Affairs in Mid-Life II: Practical Considerations

IS THERE A GOOD WAY TO HAVE AN AFFAIR?

Although it appears that some people manage their affairs better than others, when all things are considered, there may be no really good way to have an affair. Nonetheless, this question keeps arising. I have been coming to the view that should a person decide to have an affair, it ought to be done in a certain manner—a manner that keeps the partner's suspicion and awareness out of it. The person having the affair is entirely responsible for this difficult task. To have an affair well, one must be skillfully deceitful and capable of bearing the guilt within oneself.

Spouses usually become suspicious because of their perceptions that the partner is talking less, away more, increasingly irritable, has less sexual interest, and suddenly is daydreaming. The concerned spouse asks, "What is happening?" The answer is an artless dodge, "I'm just working too hard" or "Nothing is different."

A spouse's new anxiety, jealousy, suspicion, increased alcohol consumption, or depression is evidence that the person is not succeeding in having an affair the good way. The emotional decompensation has begun and it soon will be compounded by further hurtful lies, which one day culminate in "Not only did you deceive me with *that* person, but when I was suffering and did not understand why, you willfully allowed my pain to continue! You sacrificed me to your comfort!"

The person who mismanages the affair faces enormous dilemmas. A man I know confessed to his spontaneously ended affair and has spent the 3 years since listening to his pained wife return to the subject. He gave this advice to his trusted long-term friends, "One thing I now know, never, under any circumstances, *never* confess to an affair!" A patient of mine had a making-do relationship with a man after realizing that her husband had been repeatedly unfaithful in a just-sex fashion. When her husband discovered her exciting dalliance, he became desperately suicidal. The point is that affairs carry a certain danger. It may be that if one cannot have an affair in a good way, it may be wise not to have one at all.

THE MENTAL HEALTH PROFESSIONAL'S DIFFERENTIAL DIAGNOSIS

There are only a few matters that require immediate diagnostic attention.

1. Does this affair spring from a psychiatric disorder that may be thought of as impairing good judgment? If so, what is it? Is it adequately being treated?
2. Does this affair spring from some of the person's character traits? What are they?
3. Is the person dealing with the array of emotions stimulated by the affair in some diagnosable problematic way that requires attention, such as substance abuse or psychophysiological disorder?

OTHER IMPORTANT CLINICAL ASSESSMENTS

1. Is this person capable of managing the affair without threatening the viability of the family and their individual mental health?
2. What are some of the most likely short-term consequences of the extramarital behavior?

3. Can I learn something from my countertransference reactions to this particular affair? Jealousy, admiration, excitement, identification, disapproval?

PROFESSIONAL DANGERS

Sometimes many psychodynamically oriented clinicians experienced with individual psychotherapy seek to explain the affair in terms of a repetition from some past trauma. Here are some often heard explanations: repeating one's father's infidelity, dealing with one's oedipal excitement, inability to deal with the unconscious oedipal implications of marriage, childhood sexual abuse, family traditions of chaos, preoedipal attachment anxiety and distrust, replacement for mother who died when the individual was young, replacement for the emotionally distant father. Although any of these forces may be mentally operative, overemphasizing them tends to mislead the patient in two ways.

The first errant implication is that the unconscious mind generated the affair. One, therefore, does not have control or responsibility. The patient, however, already knows how the affair was initiated and maintained through various steps. The patient knows the history better than the therapist.

The second errant implication is that the therapist can help me repair this by not facing the truth, by going along with the irresistible impulse explanation. Of course, patients might reach the conclusion that they are wasting their time with this therapist.

Psychotherapists who specialize in couple's work tend to have different initial explanations for extramarital sexual involvements, but ultimately they return to childhood for the most powerful explanations.[9] These explanations for affairs emphasize the state of the marital relationship. Couples committed to amiability who are afraid of discussing anything disagreeable generate an affair to end the pattern of conflict avoidance. Other couples who feel the vulnerability inherent in deep psychological intimacy have affairs to avoid being close; they reestablish their chaotic childhood patterns in the early years of their marriage in this way. Men and women who are sexually addicted are trying to fill up their emptiness in a fruitless search to soothe their abused child within. Their codependent marriages have long been emotionally empty except for children and social activities. Although conflict avoiders, intimacy avoiders, and codependent-addicted relationships tend to be recognized in young adulthood, the empty nest affairs are middle-aged solutions to loveless devitalized marriages. Some middle-aged affairs are designed to provoke the aggrieved spouse to end the marriage, something that the unfaithful one does not have the courage to do.

In such well-intentioned schemes to organize these marital complexities into helpful categories, the therapist is the meaning-maker. It is not that such schemas do not contain cogent observations and useful descriptions; rather it is that the work of the therapist is to understand the patient's meanings first, not superimpose scientific-sounding ones. Various forms of sexual acting out, after all, are very common, if not nearly universal, private temptations. By the time clinicians are called in for some people's marital situations, it is difficult to separate the cause of the affair from the consequences of it.

EXTRAMARITAL SEX THAT MORE DIRECTLY REFLECTS LONGSTANDING PSYCHOPATHOLOGY

Some patterns of extramarital involvement indicate the presence of chronic difficulties rooted in earlier developmental disturbances. These include: compulsive sexual behavior syndromes; inability to have sex with a valued partner though readily attracted to others; paraphilia; repeated infidelity from early in marriage; attractions that are limited to married or socially unavailable men or women. When patients with these patterns are encountered in their middle years, the strains and stresses of their mid-life psychological dilemmas are not highly relevant to the understanding of the extramarital involvements. If the person is unwilling to consider the extramarital sex as a longstanding solution for old developmental problems, I have trouble believing that therapy will ultimately prove helpful. Even if the person is willing, however, such longstanding patterns are difficult to reverse, even when they are understood.

Vignette One: Sexual Compulsivity in a Paraphiliac Alcoholic

I am a bit amazed that this man is still better 7 months after I met him. A semiliterate tradesman who has been a binge drinker for over 40 years, he had failed 12 treatment attempts to gain sobriety. He was referred to me from an inpatient service where he finally acknowledged his other problem: compulsive exhibitionism. He was given ReVia (naltrexone) as a new treatment for his alcoholism. Immediately the patient noticed a "miraculous absence of craving for a drink." By early adolescence, when he began to sporadically exhibit himself, his other behaviors would have qualified him for a diagnosis of a psychopathic personality. Both of his parents and his older brother were chronic alcoholics. When inebriated 2 years ago, his brother almost died in a carbon monoxide suicide attempt.

My patient had exhibited himself to 13- and 14-year-old girls three times a week since his early 20s. Although he had been caught once, his lawyer had gotten him off without a trial and without his wife learning about this. A father of two children who was rarely home, he had not had sex with his wife for several years. Another psychiatrist, who confessed not knowing much about exhibitionism, had tried various medications for the problem but not antiandrogenic substances. I immediately placed him on 60 mg medroxyprogesterone acetate daily. Within a few days, he experienced a marked decrease in his urge to exhibit and an increase in his confidence about his ability to control his urges. He is pleased to take it, but has kept all of his contacts with me and the medication I prescribe a secret from his wife. After 4 months, he exhibited himself at a swimming pool. I added 10 mg Paxil, which seemed to give him a bit more control. During the sessions, he tells me about his tactics for self-control. I ask many questions about his work, his childhood, his hoodlum days, his courtship. He is pleased to share his history but without being asked, he does not know what to say. I think that he has not been with a doctor who has been as interested in his life history as I have been. He likes to see me. I like to see him, but infrequently; he teaches me about what passes for normal in some families.

His sexual relationship with his wife has returned. She teases him that he was having an extramarital affair that must be over now, but they both feel a lot better about his newly found time to be with his family at home. They frequently have to cope with the substance abuse of her mother, a nurse who was fired for stealing opiates. The mother-in-law, whom they rely on for childcare, is hospitalized about six times a year for a few days to dry out.

Well, it has been a pretty good month. I have not acted out but I'm worried because the weather is turning nice and there are more opportunities. I like the medications and never miss a dose. How long can I stay on them?

A long time.

I'm real busy at work. I hired a new estimator who is well known in the area and has already increased the number of jobs we have to do. It is good that I am so busy; less time for temptation.

Did you purchase the horse that you were talking about last session?

Not yet, but I still think it is a good idea. My kids are in favor of it, but my wife is not certain that I will use it enough to justify the expense. I can teach the kids how to ride, it is the one thing I think I can teach them. I had plenty of good times, you know, when I was a teenager galloping through the parks.

What about the opportunities to expose yourself in the park while riding? Do you think this will just add another temptation?

I hope not, I'll be with the kids. The place where I'm planning to keep the horse is not near the highly used portion of the park. I did used to expose myself on my horse.

You know that I have been concerned that you might exhibit to your daughter's friends.

Me, too, but so far so good. No drinking, and no exhibiting since that time at the pool. I try to avoid being around my daughter and her friends for this very reason.

Good.

WHY ARE AFFAIRS SO THREATENING?

I have long considered the answer to this question to be obvious. Ironically, my answers have changed as I have gotten older. Now my answer is that affairs threaten the structure of our lives. They rearrange our individual psyches, our relationships, our children's psyches, and the developmental trajectory of our future.

Threats to Partners

Affairs threaten us with abandonment. They assault our identity. They show us that we cannot control our destiny, let alone our partner. They confront us with the fact that our future is not certain. They humble us by quickly demonstrating to us that our planned sequence for our life is not going to occur. Affairs assault us much like death does, but death is public, inevitable, and generally carries little shame with it. Affairs convey, however erroneously, personal failure as if the betrayed one caused the partner to decide and implement the new relationship.

Affairs are long remembered. Even if they are rarely mentioned, they are not forgotten. They are part of our history as a couple. When other issues are discussed heatedly years later, the again aggrieved person may bring it up. But more importantly, when affairs are ended for the sake of the marriage, a period of private grief occurs. If it is the woman, for instance, who has been having the affair, her husband is not likely to have a large capacity to remain sympathetic to her as she recalls the sweet experiences of the past and feels sad for her loss. Of course, it is exactly the same if it is the man who has been having the affair. For women who have been betrayed, it is probably easier to bear a husband's affair that seems in her last analysis to be just-sex or make-do sex. "Did you love her?" might initially provoke a storm, "How in the world could you do that if you did not love her?" On the other hand, his "No" answer enabled him to leave the "fling" without grief and pay more concentrated attention to the wife and making their lives better.

---

* I have written this section relying heavily on the first person to emphasize the universality of the temptation to an affair and so as not to disguise human vulnerability behind professional prose.

Affairs are often the prelude to divorce in part because the feelings, attitudes, and concerns that they generate in both members of the couple are beyond their capacities to work through and master. Even when therapists are called in, divorce frequently may ensue. Divorce puts all parties on a new developmental trajectory, filled with uncertainties that cause almost all persons, however inherently mentally well, considerable anxiety, guilt, and regret. If we could separate the effects of affairs per se from the effects of divorce, perhaps we might be able to think more clearly about this subject. The trouble is that swirling within the emotional upheaval induced by the knowledge of a spousal affair are the reactions to a potential divorce.

For Middle-Aged Women and Homosexual Men

For women in mid-life, their husbands' affairs threaten them with the possibility of being alone for the rest of their lives. Many middle-aged men's affairs are with younger women. This often induces a sense of utter defeat. "How do I compete with a woman 15 years younger?" These women are not exaggerating the composition of new relationships of many divorcing middle-aged men—he 55, she 39; he 47, she 33; he 59, she 45. Do recall our discussion concerning the sexual effects of the perimenopausal years. And when gay couples break up over another man, it is typically for a younger man. When middle-aged lesbians break up over an affair, a younger woman is often involved.

What is going on here? Here are some options:

1. Aging is frightening—the younger partner helps men to deceive themselves that their age does not matter.
2. One's sexual life is perceived to be too soon over—the partner represents one more, perhaps a last, opportunity.
3. The sexual decline of mid-life is frightening—the youthfulness of the new partner provides more visual and tactile stimulation than the perimenopausal familiar one.
4. The man wants to be with a partner who is naive in the appraisal of his character; he wants to begin anew with someone who thinks highly of him.
5. The man wants to be helpful to someone whose current life issues with which he feels familiar enable him to feel more pow-

erful and competent as a companion—"Tarzan will help you, dear!"
6. All of the above.

The Gay Husband

When a wife has to deal with her husband's affair with a man as he rediscovers his homoerotic nature, she often feels in an extremely awkward circumstance. How do I compete with a man? Is he going to leave me, stay with me and be unfaithful, or stay with me forever longing for his private desire in a way that I can never compete with? Do I have AIDS? Will I get the disease if I stay with him? After all of these good years together, is his right to pursue his desire to love and be loved by a man more important than my desire not to enter into the realm of the divorced? Do I have the right to tell my friends, family, or children about why he has left or does his wish for not being known as a homosexual person supersede my needs? I love him, I know he loves me in his relatively asexual way. What am I to do?

Vignette Two from a Psychotherapy Session

A nattily dressed 60-year-old man (Ed) and his attractive 58-year-old wife (Beth) nervously came to see me after she discovered his 10-year sexual relationship with a young man. After the priest, Ed found his way to me. The couple and I worked together to preserve the relationship as the familiar story unfolded. We dealt with their emotions associated with the discovery, their desire to preserve the marriage, the thoughts and feelings that emerged after the crisis passed and more of the past was unearthed, particularly his indifference to her deteriorating mental condition. His struggles over his homoeroticism were discussed repeatedly: a few homosexual experiences in high school and college followed by shame, religiosity, and hope that he would outgrow his "immaturity"; his immersion in marriage, childrearing, and career; periodic forays to the bookstore for anonymous sex beginning in his late 40s because he felt that he had suppressed "this thing" long enough. A decade ago, however, he had met at the bookstore a 25-year-old who immediately was interested in him personally. The man had "an irresistible combination of intense desire and sexual pleasure in me." Their sexual behavior occurred within the limits of Ed's availability, but they talked almost daily.

Ed's sexual interest in Beth quickly disappeared. She remained uncertain what had happened to her marriage and grew progressively unconfident about herself. She sought help for her first episode of depression from her internist, but the few medications prescribed did not help. She tried to rationalize the mysterious loss of sexual activity to their growing older—her less attractive state and his diminished sexual desire. He gave her no reason to think he was interested in another woman and she never suspected that her husband's homoeroticism had returned, even though in courtship he once told her about his few high school experiences. As her pleasant unintimate relationship progressed during her 50s, she lost interest in her business and had to discipline herself to concentrate on her children and grandchildren. Periodic visits to different counselors never engaged her hope or stimulated a recovery.

"It had little to do with you, Beth. I've always been grateful to be married to you. It has to do with me and my attractions. He desired me and I could not resist." And the sex? "Well we had some, oral, what can I say, I don't think I can talk about it."

I often provided the words for this couple—I helped her express her rage, I helped him see the conundrum he put them into, I helped him to articulate his conundrum, and I encouraged both of them to continue to share, rather than shirk from, the many dimensions of the problem. They began making love again, this time with an intensity that neither could remember since their early marriage. Every session brought some new relevation. "It's over" was not really true nor was "he was only man." The relief from his guilt that was stated at the end of most of our sessions never lasted because, "I continued to lie about something."

The wife was a very bright eager-to-learn person who did her homework about the issue and became an accomplished sleuth. She found out who the other man was, where he lived, who he lived with, and where he worked. She skillfully exposed her husband's illusion that he was the young man's only sex partner. "Ed, you are either lying, living in lalaland, or both!" After repeated requests, I finally agreed to have him come alone to talk more freely about his situation with the man. We all anticipated the consequence of moving to weekly individual sessions: Beth would miss our sessions because they were always about the dilemmas that each of them faced, the feelings that each of them had, and the dangers that lay ahead. She decided that she was ready because she understood a great deal now and he seemed to need it. I had previously sent her to another psychiatrist to help her with her symptoms of depression, but although he knew the story, she did not feel the relief from talking to him alone that she felt talking together.

Beth asked me if I missed having sex with him. I said, "It is over, I try not to think about that anymore. Of course, I don't miss it, I put it out of my mind."

Do you think Beth believed you?

She seemed to accept it; we went on to some other subject. She asks me every day whether he called and I tell her when he does. I am no longer as afraid of what he might do. He threatened to break my windshield a long time ago; things have not been going well with his job lately and I'm afraid to tell him that I don't want him to call again. He told me that he better never catch me at the bookstore again—it is one thing to go back to your wife, but look out if you are with another man!

You always speak about your relationship like it is all him. I can't recall your saying that you don't want to give him up. But it is clear to me that you get something valuable from his phone calls, even though you don't meet him anymore.

Well, you are right about that, doctor. I like it so much that he desires me. I'm 60 years old and this young man wants to see me, have sex with me, hear about what is happening to me. He tells me that he has some sort of father thing. He likes to have sex with older men, I guess.

This is what Beth has been trying to tell you. She understands your situation. She hears you say such things like, "the only reason I don't tell him to never call again is I am afraid of what destructive thing that he might do to me." She thinks that either you are lying to her or to yourself. Beth is really aware of the nuances of this situation. You know in most of our other sessions she was explaining things to you.

I know that you are right but how can I tell her that I don't want to give up the pleasure of his desiring me?

Well, look. She asked you if you missed the sex with him. How could you NOT miss sex with this man? You told me about the intensely pleasurable "lunches" that you two had for years. You told her that you had sex with him many times. Beth had intensely pleasurable sex with you for over 25 years. SHE missed it for 10 years. She is relieved that you have resumed sex and she understands that it resumed because you two were emotionally intimate during those early months of therapy. Beth knows you now; she is aware that you have had 45 years of homoerotic desire. She just wants you to tell her the truth about what you are going through. She appreciates that you must be grieving for him or at least missing something about him.

It is so hard. It would hurt her if she believed that I miss his desire for me.

But you are still cheating on her. Once a week, he calls you, tells you about his need for you and probably excites himself on the phone.

How did you know? Sometimes he masturbates.

Oh, Ed. This is not some rare experience unique to your life. But that is not the key point. The major point is that you are still not honest with Beth and as a consequence you are setting yourself and her up for a big fall. She is only asking you to be honest, to do what you say you have done, and to not make a fool of her again.

I feel guilty all the time. I'm more honest than I used to be, but I'm still not really completely so.

I don't think this is how to do it. I'll see you next week.

For Middle-Aged Heterosexual Men

Men become highly symptomatic from their wives' affairs. Although emotional issues are essentially the same as for women, men may think that they have been particularly humiliated by the affair. Men who are cuckolds think that others are laughing at them. Their idea that there is something unique about their intense embarrassment reflects how little they appreciate what any betrayed person experiences.

What are often different are the coping opportunities. Men do not often have friends who can listen to them, or help them process what has occurred to them. They usually do not associate with other men in the same position. Men are not used to relating in this way. They tend to turn inward, drink or abuse substances, overwork, and pretend that they feel better and are functioning better than they are. The alienation that they had from their inner experiences earlier in their lives reaches a crisis point: Either they return to it, hiding their emotional realities from themselves or others, or they surrender to the profound sadness, anxiety, and anger and allow this painful experience to assist their maturation. Although some try to replace their wives, many others begin making-do relationships that tide them over until they can regain their internal sense of themselves.

Summary

Regardless of their sex, orientation, or situation, the betrayed try hard to make the best of these undesired mid-life restructurings. Because affairs restructure couples' lives whether they stay together or divorce, all involved spouses try to find the new opportunities that come from the disappointments. For women it is developing their independence, a new sense of self-sufficiency, and pleasure in exercising freedom of self-determination. For men, it is doing better this time with psychological intimacy and being less self-absorbed so that they can experience and stay in love. Affairs probably create long-term casualties of many whose capacities to forge maturation from trauma is limited. Attaining these developmental tasks may be easier to accomplish for some by divorcing, for others by staying married. For some people, the discovery of an affair is the beginning of psychiatric care (which has been shown in studies to be a factor that promotes a better outcome[1]); for others in equal need of it, it is the beginning of years of unseen anguish.

Threats to Those Who Initiated the Affair

Although the culture is used to thinking of the aggrieved spouse as the victim of the sexual acting, affairs are threatening to those who initiated them. These individuals often painfully discover their naivete.[2] They underestimated so much: their ambivalence about the new lover; the difficulty in repairing the original relationship; how deeply they hurt their partner; how their children reacted to the changes in the family and in the parent who was betrayed; how difficult it was managing two relationships; how their social world responded to them. In short, they discover that they have been foolish. This discovery may stimulate their emotional growth, but not before they have some painful soul-searching about how wrong they have been on so many accounts. This process more readily inspires humility than self-confidence.

One of the greatest dangers of an affair is to end up being surprised and disappointed by the new partner. While the affair is fresh, the problems within the marriage seem intolerable and insurmountable. The improvement that they were seeking in their lives— a fresh start with an improved partner—leads many to delay realizing the limitations that the new partner brings to the new life. Having created a tumult in the family while searching for more personal happiness, the person and the new partner often have painfully intense relationships to contend with. They need each other's help a great deal at this stage. "My (ex-) wife (husband) called today wanting...." How such mundane experiences are dealt with is crucial to the new relationship.

One may not be able to fairly judge the character of the new partner in the face of such predictable tension, but coping with the former family is part of the new couple's reality. It is a new developmental task that will not go away. Each partner is appraised by the other in terms of how the new family relationships are evolving. Some break up at this point, others succumb to despair, others proceed to make the best of it and focus on the reasons why the affair was begun in the first place.

I have not encountered too many thoughtful individuals of either sex or orientation who remain a strong advocate of affairs after their own. But I have met a few who continue to think that, despite the pain, the opportunity to have a better love relationship is worth it.

But....

Vignette Three: "What Are We Going to Do?"

Let's say a successful, robustly healthy man gradually grows impotent too young in mid-life and realizes, after much anguish, that his mysterious lack of desire and potency are unmistakably related to his inability to be psychologically intimate with his loved, respected, and much-enjoyed wife. An emerging relationship with a seemingly happily married middle-aged woman with children clarifies his enigmatic problems. She is determined to persist in their evolving highly pleasurable friendship. He sees that she likes their closeness, impotent or not. Their easy exchange of feelings about the many facets of their lives helps him to understand that he and his wife are formal, polite, sensitive to each other's social and vocational needs, and good problem solvers, but not intimate with each other. His potency and desire slowly recovers, but not for his wife. On both relationship fronts, he and his partner struggle with the question, "What are we going to do?" He and his friend know that they do not want to stop. They both choose to stay married—for their spouses, themselves, and the progression of their lives with their children and grandchildren. They rework their concept of themselves as honest people; we still are but not about this. If a partner ever asks, "Are you having an affair?" they have decided to lie so as not to hurt the partner. Better this than wreck two families. Both recognize the wish to run off and be together forever, but they decide to tolerate their deceit.

"What are we going to do?" is a matter that the spouses discuss too. She knows that her husband has been to doctors to no avail. She sees that he is trying to make love but fails to erect and feels badly. The wife is kindly silent, does not initiate sex, and continues to be appreciative of what they do have together. She keeps her thoughts of her husband having another woman to herself. Thankfully, they are now more tired at night than they were a few years ago. Each remembers that they had a good sex life for the first 30 years—even without psychological intimacy. Can this situation endure? For how long? Until when?

Why do people take such risks? For the opportunity to experience a love that is both fresh and seems to contain a greater potential to more fully realize the ideals of love. By mid-life, long marriages have declared their strengths and weaknesses. Each partner has to accept the limitations. Affairs may be the rebellion against this acceptance—a private social hedge against acceptance. It is not merely a male gender strategy.

Vignette Four: "I Want to Have a Sex Life"

A middle-aged career woman in her second marriage now has lovely children with a fine man who has managed to not have sexual behavior with her for several years. No explanations have been offered for his marriage-long low interest in sex, but he will "do better just as soon as this work problem is over, etc." A married man from out of town expresses interest. Soon her sexual desert vanishes. Convenient. He is in town occasionally. They have wonderful but abbreviated evenings, and it is back to their separate lives. They communicate several times a week through their pagers. The only problem is that talk starts at their workplace. He gets frightened and withdraws for a while. She, who prides herself on self-control, feels uneasily sad and on the early edge of desperate. She has grown to really like him, miss him, and repeatedly thinks about how nice it would be to live with a man who is attracted to her sexually. This was such a nice solution. "I had my sexual life, it was just not with my husband. I thought for many years that I was not the type of person who did such things but I was surprised how readily I responded and how little guilt I felt. Oh well, now I have a secret too. My husband is keeping one either from himself or me—why he does not want to make love."

A little time passes, and they meet again. This time they realize that they have grown to depend on this and do not want it to end. "What are we going to do?"

Ah! The familiar question.

ARE AFFAIRS HOMOGENEOUS?

From the biases inherent in clinical work, the answer to this question is "Yes, in a dangerous way." They all result from a personal decision to initiate or allow someone else's initiation to proceed. They all are potentially dangerous to the immediate and extended family members. They change a couple's relationship, often, not invariably, for the worse. They change each person's psyche—the betrayed and the betrayer. Affairs are the difficult road to travel—the road of imagined solutions that carry an unerasable risk of creating more problems than they solve.

It is not just younger people who do not quite realize the power of genital union to generate emotional bonds. Having an affair, even one of such convenience, knowing from the beginning that neither is interested in changing partners, has the potential to educate people about how human attachment can operate.

REFERENCES

1. Kaffman, M. Divorce in the kibbutz: Lessons to be drawn. *Family Process* 32:117–132, 1993.
2. Parks, T. Adultery: Why settle for a marriage that is less than perfect? *The New Yorker* June 24, 1996, pp. 128–132.

The Sexual Side Effects of Serotonergic Antidepressant Medications

THE WHISPERING MAN

When 42-year-old Bill was given paroxetine for his prolonged mysterious bout of anxious depression without hypomania, the drug seemed to organize a speedy complete recovery within 6 weeks. Another psychiatrist had successfully treated him with a tricyclic antidepressant for his two previous depressions. The patient immediately preferred the seemingly side-effect-less paroxetine. As he gradually returned to his normal state, he shyly whispered to me that the only difficulties with this wonderful drug—and "believe me, doctor, they really are not problems"—were that he now lasted longer during intercourse and sometimes could not ejaculate. I explained to him that this symptom was related to the medication and that many individuals experience such difficulty, "some transiently." At this stage, both he and his wife of 21 years were delighted that he was once again enjoying his children and running his small business without his paralyzing worries, social withdrawal, and "I just don't feel good" explanations. Although sexually functional while depressed, he lacked enthusiasm for everything including sex. At our half-hour follow-up visits when I intended to better understand the psychological sources of his depression, sexual side effects were always the first and sometimes the only matters about which we spoke. His voice always softened when he spoke about sex. I had to catch myself from responding to him sotto voce. During a subsequent visit, he gently explained that he was still having problems ejaculating, then suddenly losing his whisper, he said that "it does not seem to matter to me. This is so curious because sex has always been an important part of my life." Their sexual frequency had diminished from eight to two times a month.

From our earliest contacts I had been emphasizing that his third episode of depression meant to me that he should indefinitely take an antidepressant to prevent or attenuate the severity of a fourth episode. After 9 months of feeling well, he informed me that there was another side effect that he did not like, in fact, that frightened him. "I seem indifferent to too many things. For instance, I used to cry at movies and now I am not moved. Maybe the reason I got better from my depression was that the medicine stopped allowing me to care about my business problems and fears of going bankrupt like my father did. I'm worried what I'm becoming." By this time, I had already reduced his dose of paroxetine, given him weekend holidays, further reduced his weekly dosage, and added yohimbine—all to no avail. We rediscussed two options for his consideration: (1) discontinuing paroxetine entirely and enduring the risk of a return of symptoms or (2) changing medications. I was hesitant about both options. By the next visit, he had already implemented the first plan and, within 4 days, he began having 2- to 4-second episodes of dizziness. This withdrawal symptom cleared up 8 hours after taking 10 mg of the drug. He decided to stay on paroxetine for a while longer.

The Effect on the Wife

His wife had been orgasmic during most of their sexual experiences. Now that he was obviously long over his depression, she did not like the fact that he often could not reach orgasm. She told him that she felt too selfish being taken care of sexually when she could not please him. With great effort he occasionally ejaculated but the effort discouraged both of them from having sex again soon. The whispering man did not talk easily about sex even with his wife. As his relative anorgasmia and drivelessness continued, she could not quite believe that a medication could diminish her husband's interest in sex. Her initial understanding attitude gave way to impatience which was in turn replaced by agitation and argumentativeness in a way that he had never seen before. When he angrily shouted (uncharacteristically) in exasperation, "Why the hell are you so crabby lately?" she told him. "I know you are seeing another woman! Why else would my young, healthy, always sexually eager husband lose interest?" After calling me for advice to help in calming her down, we agreed that he should ask her to accompany him to our next visit so that I could try to reassure her. I had planned to explain to her that other people have lost their sexual drive with the (then) three newer antidepressants. But her intense anxiety and suspiciousness dissipated during the next week as his visit drew near and she did not arrive with her husband. "Believe me, doctor, it was a week from hell dealing with her."

A Reminder about the Sexual Equilibrium

Although the antisexual impact of modern antidepressants has become much better known in the last several years,[1] what is not commonly appreciated is the effect of these sexual changes on the sexual equilibrium. Physicians tend to think about side effects only in terms of their individual patients. But, as explained in Chapter 5, partnered sexual life occurs within a matrix of two people's interconnected psychologies. Partners notice the changing sexual component characteristics of their mates and regard them in some way. Their regard may be positive or negative but always gives rise to a personal interpretation of what is transpiring. The partners' interpretations may not make sense to therapists because they do not have the same information that the partners have. No matter how much we know about our patients, their partners may know their histories more completely, may link the current sexual deficits to other life events differently, and may arrive at a separate conclusion. The whispering man's wife seemed paranoid to me about what was to me an obviously medication-induced sexual dysfunction.

The Wife's Other Knowledge

As the patient and I were considering this turn of events, I recalled that he had once told me about his wife's disfiguring labia majora and minora surgery a year ago. Other than the initial worry about cancer, he seemingly had put the matter out of his mind. However, he had recently formed a friendship with a younger cousin. Although his wife knew about the friendship, she had no inkling of his growing sexual fantasies about the cousin. Perhaps the whispering man was still whispering when he spoke of sex because of his escalating erotic preoccupation with his cousin. Perhaps his friendship with his cousin was partially motivated by his need to energize his fading sexual capacities. Perhaps his wife was deeply worried about the impact of her vulvar surgery on her husband's sexual desire. Perhaps she separately worried about what was going on between this long lost young relative and the renewed friendship with her husband at their lunch meetings.

Despite his private excitement over another woman and their serious contemplation of an affair, I considered his new sexual dysfunction as an ordinary example of a selective serotinergic reuptake inhibitor (SSRI)-induced problem. He did not feel guilty about the contemplated affair; he just wanted to discuss it so he could make up his mind. He decided against it. In all of these discussions he whispered.

The whispering man's organic sexual dysfunction generated a new psychological force within himself and his wife that led to her transient change in behavior. This is how the sexual equilibrium operates—conscious and not so conscious factors influence both partners' psychology.

TOWARD A PERSPECTIVE ON SEXUAL SIDE EFFECTS

The Sophistication of Modern Psychopharmacology

Modern psychopharmacology has impressively advanced methodologically in its ability to scientifically establish the efficacy of medications for psychiatric conditions. This highly refined scientific know-how is necessary to gain Food and Drug Administration (FDA) approval for a new drug or a new indication for an already approved drug. These methods include care in selection of the patients reflected in defined inclusion and exclusion criteria; randomization; doubleblindedness; placebo control; standardized outcome assessments; independent assessment team; large sample sizes involving multiple sites and investigators; sophisticated data analyses; and sometimes crossover designs or head-to-head comparison of one standard antidepressant with the new candidate for the prescription market. More than one sophisticated study is always necessary to establish a medication as useful. As a result of these expensive processes, physicians now have a wide variety of modern medications to use for the common problems of depressive and anxiety disorders.

The use of such stringent methods has been evolving as clinical pharmacology has advanced. There are specialists in study design who, although working for a pharmaceutical firm that has a strong financial interest in a favorable study result, are able to set up protocols that can be expected to objectively answer a question about a drug's utility for a condition. Not all of these experts in study design work in the drug manufacturing industry. Many work in academic centers and others for the National Institute of Mental Health and the FDA itself. Considerable expertise in study design and interpretation abounds.

The FDA has not yet required a scientific monitoring of the sexual side effects of drugs in development for psychiatric or medical conditions. So the incidence figures reported on this topic from pre-FDA approval studies generally reflect only the patients who spontaneously mentioned these effects. Once a drug is on the market, side effects that may not have shown up in the earliest studies, are generally left to the practicing physician to deal with. The pharmaceutical industry is far from indifferent to the emerging side effect problem. Companies are often supportive in funding educational workshops to consider the problem. Other companies seeing the sexual side effect problem perceive an opportunity to develop new products with similar antidepressant efficacy without sexual side effects. Other companies see an opportunity to increase their share of the lucrative antidepressant market by educating the medical public about the low incidence of sexual side effects with their long-existent product. They may even fund a sophisticated study to demonstrate their product's pattern of preserving sexual function. These are the routine dynamic competitive market forces at work that subtly vie for the physician to prescribe their product as long as they retain the exclusive patent on their medication.

The Range of Sexual Problems Attributed to Antidepressants

In the meantime, we have depressed patients like the whispering man who often become fully or partially better from the basic psychiatric condition but develop sexual side effects.[2] Although the tricyclic antidepressants and certainly the monoamine oxidase inhibitors were known to sometimes interfere with sexual functioning, they never earned the reputation that the first generation of SSRIs acquired by the mid-1990s.[3] Results of studies vary in the extent to which fluoxetine, sertraline, and paroxetine produce sexual difficulties. Men generally are thought to complain more about them than women, but the explanation for this may be more psychosocial than pharmacological.

Men

The sexual symptoms of men that have been attributed to use of the SSRIs include (asterisks indicate the more common symptoms):

- Difficulty attaining orgasm*
- Burning during and after ejaculation
- Inability to ejaculate or attain orgasm*
- Penile anesthesia
- Difficulty obtaining or sustaining an erection
- Diminished sexual drive*
- Prolonged erection or priapism
- Decreased pleasure of orgasm

Women

The sexual symptoms of women that have been attributed to use of the SSRIs include (asterisks indicate the more common symptoms):

- Vaginal and clitoral anesthesia
- Inefficient or unsustainable arousal
- Difficulty and delay in attaining orgasm*
- Inability to attain orgasm*
- Diminished sexual drive*
- Clitoral tumescence

- Clitoral tumescence followed by orgasm in response to yawning
- Decreased pleasure of orgasm

The Basic Questions

Physicians need to know how various antidepressants negatively and positively influence sexual function, that is, the specific neuro-chemical mechanism involved. To what extent do these mechanisms take place in the brain, spinal cord, and genitals? Where in the brain? Why is there a different time course for orgasmic inhibition (very quick), antidepressant effect (weeks), and drive reduction (weeks to months)? Why are some people unaffected by sexual side effects? The driving force behind these questions is the need to learn how to prevent or minimize sexual dysfunction. Antidepressant-induced sexual problems, however, provide an excellent opening to understand the biological substrate of human sexual dysfunction.

In terms of the usual research complexities that academic mental health professionals deal with, the issue is relatively simple because it is only biological.[4] Biological problems are far more suitable to scientific unraveling than psychodynamic matters of psychological causality and rehabilitation.

What Studies Are Needed

For starters, the field needs a series of prospective accounts of the incidence of each sexual side effect stratified by patients' age, sex, psychiatric diagnosis, and antidepressant used. The studies should describe the baseline prevalence of the sexual dysfunctions that existed prior to the depression and during the depression prior to pharmacotherapy. They should then characterize when and at what dosage level the symptoms appeared, their degree (mild, moderate, and severe), their course without intervention (spontaneously resolved, remained the same, worsened, fluctuated), the sexual context being affected (masturbation, partner sex), and the response to physician interventions.

The interpretation of such a set of studies will be confounded by three additional matters. First, the medications may enhance people's sexual life because they effectively treat the psychiatric condition that has limited them in so many subtle ways. Patients and their doctors may be confused because sexual life can both improve ("I enjoy it more now") and become different ("I just cannot reach orgasm"). This is more likely to be the case for women because women are used to a less reliable arousal and orgasmic experience. Second, when drugs are introduced, because of the cost of performing studies, their efficacy is usually based on experiences with depressed persons over relatively short periods of up to 3 months. If sexual side effects emerge after longer periods of the medication use, the actual incidence may be significantly underappreciated. Some of these new studies have to be longer. Third, the medications may in some people enhance sexual function directly—biologically. At this stage, sexual enhancement by the SSRIs should not be counted on by patients and their physicians; it is, however, an intriguing matter that gets more mention in the literature than its incidence would otherwise dictate because of the deep human interest in enhancing sexual response through aphrodisiacs (recently renamed *prosexual agents*).

The Irony

The irony is that working out of these questions is largely left to the practicing physician whose skills generally do not include a high degree of sophistication in study design. Clinicians' research tend to be based on what they do—that is, case reports, anecdotal experiences, and a few energetic less expensive retrospective surveys of psychiatric practices.[5,6] This is the typical, early, valuable but less scientific impressionistic stage of clinical science. If the problem remains unsolved by such observations, more powerful, expensive, and sophisticated multimodal research efforts are necessary.

Current Frequency Data

It has long been established that the frequency of a sexual problem is related to how the information is collected. For instance, one study of antidepressants in the pre-SSRI era demonstrated that spontaneous report generated a 10% incidence, interview 26%, and questionnaire 47%.[7] But, it depends on the questionnaire; some are more sensitive than others.[8]

Generally, the range of orgasmic difficulties related to the SSRIs is presented as between 40 and 71%. If clomipramine is considered an SSRI, the upper limit should be stated as nearly 100%, depending on the criterion used for anorgasmia.[9] Drive deficiencies, which are listed as problems with libido, are often quoted as having a much lower incidence. Incidence figures for the other side effects are rarely provided. Here are some examples of incidence figures with various SSRIs: orgasmic delay in both sexes, 62%[10] sexual dysfunction, 43[2] sexual dysfunction among women within the first year of treatment, 45%.[12] Early data have begun to accumulate comparing one SSRI with another: Sertraline produces more dysfunction (35%) among depressed outpatients than fluvoxamine (10%).[13] Paroxetine produces slightly more sexual "problems" than sertraline and fluoxetine.[5] In some studies, however, the incidence is statistically similar and 1.6 times more likely to occur among the SSRIs than the tricyclics.[14] More recently approved antidepressants such as nefazodone (which has serotonergic activity) seem to generate far less sexual problems than the SSRIs.[15]

An improved methodological approach to the problem of the incidence of sexual dysfunction was recently published.[*] It used a systematic direct interview of 344 Spanish patients who reported normal sexual function prior to their use of fluoxetine, paroxetine, sertraline, or fluvoxamine. Fourteen percent of the patients reported sexual dysfunction spontaneously; when questiond systematically the incidence rose to 58%. There were no significant differences in the combined incidence of sexual dysfunction among the four SSRIs; the incidence figures ranged between 65% and 54%. Paroxetine generated significantly more anorgasmia and arousal difficulties (impotence and inadequate lubrication) than other SSRIs, however. Despite the sexual dysfunction, 24.5% of patients seem to well tolerate their new pattern without affecting their compliance with the regimen (12 of these were men with premature ejaculation). Men had less severe dysfunction than women

* Montejo-Gonzalez, A.L., Llorca, G., Izquierdo, J.A., Ledesma, A., Bousono, M., Calcedo, A., Carrasco, J.L., Cuidad, J., Daniel, E., De La Gandara, J., Derecho, J., Franco, M., Gomez, M.J., Macias, J.A., Martin, T., Perez, V., Sanchez, M., Sanchez, S., Vicens, E. SSRI-induced sexual dysfunction: Fluoxetine, paroxetine, sertraline, and fluvoxamine in a prospective, multicenter, and descriptive clinical study of 344 patients. *Journal of Sex and Marital Therapy* 23(3): 176–194, 1997.

but a 9% greater incidence. Older patients were more severely affected by the SSRIs.

It is important to note four related matters: (1) Few of the studies referenced above fulfill reasonably sophisticated methodological expectations; (2) incidence figures provided by the *Physician's Desk Reference* and pharmaceutical company advertising have historically vastly underestimated the incidence of sexual side effects; (3) the longer an SSRI is on the market, the more clear the sexual side effect problem has become; (4) the means of collecting incidence figures is not always specified by the authors.

The exact figures are not the major point, however. *The point is that the scientific sophistication and care with which a drug is studied to bring it to the medical marketplace is in no way matched by the efforts to characterize or ameliorate the sexual side effect problem.*

DEALING WITH SEXUAL SIDE EFFECTS

The efforts to deal with the sexual side effects of SSRIs are not yet highly funded. The following drugs have been described in the psychiatric literature as "effective" when given along with the serotonergic antidepressant in reversing the antisexual effects[15]:

- Amantadine[17]—a dopamine agonist used in doses of 100–400 mg/day
- Bupropion[18]—no effect on serotonin uptake but used in doses of 75 to 150 mg
- Buspirone[19]—thought to have an affinity for the $5HT_{1A}$ and D_2 receptors; doses begin at 5 mg.
- Cyproheptadine[20]—an antihistamine and appetite stimulant with cortical $5HT_2$ blockading properties whose use in a wide dosage range of 2 to 16 mg can induce both sedation and acute reversal of antidepressant effect[21]
- Dextroamphetamine—a dopamine agonist
- Methylphenidate[22]—a dopamine agonist
- Nefazodone[23]—thought to have more activity at $5HT_3$ receptor than SSRIs
- Yohimbine[24]—a presynaptic α_2-adrenergic antagonist whose doses range between 5.4 and 16.2 mg daily

The basis for these recommendations may have been a clinician's hunch, an understanding of the possible mechanisms of the sexual side effects, or some other astute clinical observation. This per se is fine; it is one of the ways that medicine evolves, but it is only the beginning process in establishing a clinical usefulness of an approach to a problem.

Clinicians need to be wary, however. These reports are basically anecdotal accounts of a physician trying the medication on a patient or two with the problem. If the response is an improvement by the next visit, more patients get tried on variable doses of the drug chosen to counteract the sexual side effect and a paper is presented at a meeting and subsequently reported in a newsletter. Sometimes a Letter to the Editor is generated. If the early patients do not respond positively, their doses are increased; if they still do not respond, this negative result is not typically brought to the literature. In methodological terms, the physician is conducting a single-site, open-label, or nonblinded clinical trial that does not control dose, has no separate objective quantifiable measurement, and generates no confidence in the duration of the positive clinical response, the patients' capacities to use the additional drug as a long-term solution, or the comparative efficacy of one approach versus another. When these topics are presented at continuing education meetings, the anecdotal nature of the initial observations is typically not emphasized.[25] Positive results from such crude clinical endeavors are the reasons to approach the matter with more scientific sophistication, however. In all branches of medicine, most claims from individual practitioners fail to hold up when they are tested with better methods. There, too, whenever 8 treatments have been recommended for a problem, the physician generally immediately recognizes that none of them are conspicuously effective.

Here are the reasons better methods must be employed: Open physician-prescribed trials cannot hope to separate:

- Expectation effects *from*
- Spontaneous improvement (that has already been occasionally observed) *from*
- Fluctuating effects of psychological factors in the patient's sexual equilibrium *from*
- Lies about the drug's effects told so as not to disappoint the doctor *from*

- The doctor's misinterpretation of what the patient's experience has been *from*
- A genuine pharmacologically induced physiological improvement.

The problem is that practicing physicians and their patients want to know what to do about this problem—they do not want to hear about the limitations of science. They want to try something.

Here is one other reason for caution in uncritically following the anecdotal reports of physicians: Recently, it has been reported that an over-the-counter herbal preparation, *Ginkgo biloba*, has been helpful in reversing sexual dysfunction caused by SSRIs.[10] Forty-four of fifty-two (84.6%) patients on a variety of antidepressants were helped when given 60–420 mg daily of ginkgo obtained at health foods stores in an open-label self-report observational study by one physician.[26] What was not appreciated when this approach was suggested to patients, however, was that this preparation had been reported to be the cause of a bilateral subdural hematoma in a healthy 33-year-old and spontaneous bleeding into the iris in another patient.[27] *Ginkgo biloba* seems to interfere with platelet aggregation and to prolong bleeding time!

IS IT KNOWN HOW SSRIs GENERATE SEXUAL DYSFUNCTION?

As a class, the SSRIs are often preferred by clinicians over the tricyclics for depression because of their side effect profile. This is assumed to increase medication tolerability and compliance with the physicians recommendations.[28] When compared with the less expensive tricyclic antidepressants (TCAs), the SSRIs are similarly effective and have a similar time to onset of antidepressant effects. But they generally do not produce *muscarinic* (blurred vision, dry mouth, sedation, urinary retention, constipation, arrhythmias), *histaminic* (drowsiness), and *alpha-adrenergic* (hypotension, sedation) side effects. Their most common side effects are nausea, nervousness or agitation, insomnia, and sexual ones. The TCAs and the monoamine oxidase inhibitors can produce dose-related sexual side effects as well, but these, too, are considered to be the result of the serotonergic reuptake inhibiting properties of these compounds.

The SSRIs also produce idiosyncratic side effects such as sweating, headache, diarrhea, and rash, which generally are unexplained neurophysiologically. The SSRIs are not uniform in their risk of side effects. Paroxetine has more sedation and a greater risk of withdrawal symptoms, for example, whereas fluvoxamine tends to produce nausea more often than others.[29] Although named for their dominant neurophysiological effects on measurable neurotransmission, the SSRIs actually inhibit neuronal reuptake of serotonin, noradrenaline, and dopamine. Higher doses are generally required to inhibit the reuptake of dopamine, however. These findings refer only to brain mechanisms and only to certain portions of the brain. Peripheral effects occur and may be relevant to the production of early onset sexual side effects.

For physicians who manage antidepressant side effects, knowledge of these patterns has to be sufficient to make choices for medication selection for individual patients. The physician often categorizes the patient's side effects as *serotonergic, muscarinic, alpha-adrenergic,* or *uncertain* in terms of neurotransmitter overstimulation or blockade. A decision is made as to whether the symptom is likely to be short or long term and whether the patient's cooperation and quality of life with treatment are threatened by it. This knowledge does not constitute an understanding of how SSRIs generate sexual side effects.

Another potentially helpful view of the mechanism of production derives from studies of the neurophysiology of sexual behavior in animals ranging from rats to nonhuman primates.[30] Elegant animal studies can carefully control relevant biological variables and experiment with one biological parameter at a time. Even so, biologists recognize that the sexual behavior of animals is influenced by social (dominance) and environmental factors (adequacy of food supply).

Within carefully arranged experiments, the complexity of the biological substrate of sexuality remains impressive. Sexual behavior varies from species to species in important ways and within a given species is the end product of the interaction of opposing agonist–antagonist influences. Sex is not simple for animals either or at least the understanding of how the primate nervous system generates sexual behavior is not yet known to be a straightforward matter of turning some biological switch on or off.

A brief summary of the current general thinking about sexual effects of varieties of *serotonergic, dopaminergic,* and *adrenergic* neurotransmission in the brains of rhesus monkeys follows.[31] It is offered to evoke a sense of the complexity of the biological possibilities for causing sexual dysfunction.

Serotonin—Stimulation of the $5HT_{2C}$ receptor provokes erection, increases the time to ejaculation, and increases the frequency of copulation. Stimulation of the $5HT_{1A}$ receptor does not produce erections; it does decrease the time to ejaculation, and diminishes the frequency of copulation. Using an antagonist to the $5HT_{2A}$ receptor makes ejaculation difficult.

Dopamine—When either apomorphine (a mixed D_1/D_2 receptor agonist) or quinlorane (a D_2 receptor agonist) is administered to males, erections and (in the presence of a female) masturbation are provoked. These monoamines delay the animals' ability to ejaculate and increase the frequency of their copulations. When a D_1 receptor agonist is administered, however, there are no sexual effects. When a D_1 antagonist is administered, ejaculation is inhibited.

Norepinephrine—The administration of yohimbine (a α_2-adrenergic antagonist) does not facilitate any sexual behavior in rhesus monkeys but does in stumptail monkeys. However, various α_2 compounds produce sexual effects in rhesus monkeys.

A reasonable conclusion from animal work is that the effects of the drug treatments vary greatly, depending on the neurotransmitter receptor subtype being manipulated, the dose of drug being administered, and the behavior being evaluated. Drug administration to monkeys can have a beneficial effect on a specific component of sexual behavior—erection, time to ejaculation, frequency of copulation, for instance—at one dose, and at either the same or a different dose, the drug can interfere with another component of sexual behavior. It is quite possible that different parts of the brain, spinal cord, and genital organs are influenced in opposite ways by the same drugs. The clinical implication of this research for humans, who, unlike rhesus monkeys, can talk, is that although it may be possible to use pharmacological agents to treat discrete deficits in male sexual function, it is also possible that any such treatment may compromise a different functional component of male sexual behavior. One can see why the sexual side effects of the SSRIs are thought to involve some aspect of serotonin activity. Still the questions, "What is going on?" "Where is it occurring?" remain unanswered.

Although clinicians often explain the sexual side effects of the SSRIs by stating that there is an excessive amount of serotonin at the synapse, it is clear from animal research that there are many serotonergic receptor types in the brain—12 at last count.[32] When physicians administer these drugs, there is little useful clinical understanding why one person has sexual side effects, another does not, and yet a rare other seems to have some sexual enhancement.

The Use of Yohimbine

Yohimbine, the α_2-adrenergic antagonist, is being increasingly used for many prosexual purposes, such as treating erectile dysfunction, low desire states, and SSRI-induced dysfunctions. It has been systematically studied in humans in several ways with quite variable responses. In a study using a continuous intravenous infusion of an α_2-adrenergic antagonist (not yohimbine), young nondysfunctional men but not older ones had more nocturnal non-REM erections. Even in the responsive young men, however, differing doses generated significantly different nocturnal erection responses.[33] The increased use of this drug has been impressive lately. To what extent it actually works, under what circumstances, and for how long remains to be established. When used to combat fluoxetine-induced sexual dyfunction in a non-blind fashion, eight of nine patients reported some improvement but five reported side effects; two discontinued its use.[34]

SSRIs and Middle-Aged Persons

Given the limits of information about incidence, mechanisms of production, and treatment of the sexual side effects of these drugs, we might be particularly worried about adding to the burdens of men and women in their expected sexual physiological decline in the 50s. Our worries should be focused on the patient him- or herself, the partner, and their sexual equilibrium. Raising the issue of sexual side effects before treatment is commenced creates an opportunity to find out about the current state of sexual functioning. This in turn helps to make more intelligent clinical choices.

One Clinical Algorithm

Given the deficiencies in understanding the mechanisms of production of the sexual side effects, one approach to this issue for clinicians who prescribe these medications is the following.

1. Learn each patient's sexual capacities and the importance of their sexual functioning to them prior to administering an antidepressant drug.

2. If the patient is sexually dysfunctional—in desire, arousal, orgasm, or satisfaction domains—try to ascertain whether it is related to the primary psychiatric diagnosis for which the patient is seeking treatment, a comorbid psychiatric condition, an organic factor, or a longstanding psychogenic difficulty.[35]

3. Select the antidepressant medication with the above information in mind. Although we psychiatrists like to think that about 70% of our prescriptions for an antidepressant will catalyze a significant patient improvement, psychopharmacologists now distinguish the rate of response of those who persist on medication for a full course from the rate of response of all those begun on the medication. The latter is closer to 50%. Many of those who stop taking the medication are switched to another medication with fewer side effects and they get better. Many considerations are brought to bear on the selection of an antidepressant medication—the sexual life of the patient is merely one of them. A 50-year-old divorced person, depressed since left by the spouse, frightened about closeness to anyone, who does not masturbate, and who emphatically states a lack of interest in sexual relationships, is the type of patient for whom a physician may reasonably ignore the possibility of sexual side effects.

4. Explain the problem of sexual side effects to the patient early in the treatment. Orgasm dampening effects of the SSRIs can begin within 48 hours. Prolongation of time to ejaculation is often not a problem for men and their partners. In fact, the SSRIs are now used as a treatment for premature ejaculation. Anorgasmia may vary with the degree of excitement of each sexual experience, and for some people the sexual side effects

seem to spontaneously remit.[36] Men who tend to be sexually compulsive and feel driven to behave sexually in problematic ways may particularly benefit from the reduction in sexual drive. The SSRIs, in fact, are the drugs now most commonly prescribed for people whose complaints suggest compulsive sexual behavior, namely, paraphilia, sexual addictions, and sexual obsessions. For most other patients, however, loss of drive may be a long-term problem for them, their partners, or both.

5. Lower the dose of the medication, carefully staying in touch with the patient to ascertain that the antidepressant efficacy has not been lost.

6. Try to skip the medication on the days when the patient can reasonably anticipate that partner sexual behavior is likely to occur. Drug holidays would seem to be less effective for fluoxetine because of its long-acting metabolite,[37] although this is based on a few anecdotal experiences.

7. If the patient develops significant negative sexual effects, change medication to one that is thought to have a significantly lower incidence of sexual side effects. These include nefazodone, bupropion, venlafaxine, trazodone, and tricyclics. Don't be too surprised if the patient has intolerable side effects or if the sexual symptom persists with the new medication, however. Some patients may not develop sexual side effects to the same degree with another SSRI.

8. Consider adding one of the eight drugs previously listed after discussing with the patient the possibility of side effects from adding a drug.

SEXUAL EFFECTS OF OTHER MEDICATIONS

Physicians have long been aware that psychotropics and other medications have a potential to generate sexual complaints in patients.[38] The complaints are far better known among men than women. The scientific limitations of knowledge in these areas are similar to those for the serotonergic antidepressants. The *Medical Letter* periodically publishes reviews of this topic, but these have the effect of assisting physicians to associate a drug category with desire, arousal, or orgasmic problems. The mechanisms of action are varied but often are not completely understood. The antihypertensive medications have received the most scientific attention. The cancer chemotherapeutic agents are probably the most overlooked and underinvestigated powerful inducers of sexual dysfunction.

Antihypertensive Medications

The antihypertensive agents are relatively well studied because (1) hypertension is a common illness often first diagnosed in middle age in people who otherwise feel normal; (2) two of the earliest effective antihypertensive drugs, reserpine and guanethidine, gained a reputation for generating male desire, arousal, and orgasmic dysfunctions[39]; (3) pharmaceutical companies have long been searching for compounds that have a low incidence of sexual side effects so as to increase patient compliance. Pharmaceutical research has lately been highly successful. Compared to the earliest antihypertensive agents and the generations of β-adrenergic blocking agents, the many varieties of calcium channel blocker and the ACE inhibitors represent a major advance in minimizing sexual effects. However, careful studies have demonstrated that the incidence of sexual dysfunction increases significantly in the following order: nonhypertensive men < untreated hypertensive men < hypertensive men treated with one drug < hypertensive men treated with two drugs < hypertensive men treated with three drugs.[40]

Cancer Treatments

Cancer is often treated with hormones that have sexual effects. Men with prostate cancer are often given various agents to diminish or eradicate androgen production. Agents such as diethylstilbestrol and lupron effectively diminish serum testosterone levels and slow tumor progression, but they also diminish sexual desire and limit potency. Women with estrogen receptor-positive breast cancer are now routinely treated with tamoxifen, which induces or deepens menopause and blocks the effects of estrogen on the genital urinary tract. Having a life-threatening illness per se may so disturb a person that normal sexual function becomes difficult. Men and women with cancer often are given powerful antineoplastic compounds, which may create various sexual deficits on their own. When the matter at hand is curing the person's tumor, physicians and their patients understandably pay little attention to the sexual consequences of medications.

REFERENCES

1. Demythenaere, K., and Vanderschureren, D. Selective serotonin reuptake inhibitors and sexual function. In: J. Bancroft (ed.), *The Pharmacology of Sexual Function and Dysfunction.* Excerpta Medica: Amsterdam, 1995, pp. 327–345.

2. Brodkin, J.A., Lasser, R.A., Wines, J.D., Gardner, D.M., and Baldessarini, R.J. Combining serotonin reuptake inhibitors and bupropion in partial responders to antidepressant monotherapy. *Journal of Clinical Psychiatry* 58(4):137–144, 1997.

3. Jensvold, M.F., Plaut, V.C., Rojansky, N., Crenshaw, T.L., and Halbreich, U. Sexual side effects of psychotropic drugs in women and men. In: M.F. Jensvold, U. Halbreich, and J.A. Hamilton (eds.), *Psychopharmacology and Women: Sex, Gender, and Hormones.* American Psychiatric Press: Washington, DC, 1996, pp. 323–370.

4. Aveline, M.O. The limitation of randomized controlled trials as guides to clinical effectiveness with reference to the psychotherapeutic management of neuroses and personality disorders: Editorial review. *Current Opinion in Psychiatry* 10(2):113–115, 1997.

5. Ashton, A.K., Hamer, R., and Rosen, R.C. Serotonin reuptake inhibitor-induced sexual dysfunction and its treatment: A large-scale retrospective study of 596 psychiatric outpatients. *Journal of Sex and Marital Therapy* 23(3): 165–175, 1997.

6. DeLeo, D., and Magni, G. Sexual side effects of antidepressant drugs. *Psychosomatics* 24:1076–1082, 1983.

7. Schein, M., Zyzanski, S., Levine, S.B., Dickman, R., and Alegomagno, S. The frequency of sexual problems among family practice patients. *Family Practice Research Journal* 7(3):122–134, 1988.

8. Monteiro, W.O., Noshirvani, H.F., Marks, I.M., and Lelliot, P.T. Anorgasmia from clomipramine in obsessive-compulsive disorder: A controlled trial. *British Journal of Psychiatry* 151:107–112, 1987.

9. Grimes, J.B., Labbate, L.A., and Hines, A.H. Sexual dysfunction induced by SSRIs. Presented at the 1996 American Psychiatric Association Meeting, Abstract 95.

10. Montejo, A.L., Llorce, G., and Izquierdo, J.A., Sexual dysfunction with SSRIs: A comparative analysis. Presented at the 1996 American Psychiatric Association Meeting, Abstract 717.

11. Aldrich, A.P., Cook, M.D., and Pedersen, L. Retrospective review of psychotropic-induced sexual dysfunction in women. Presented at the 1996 American Psychiatric Association Meeting, Abstract 714.

12. Nemeroff, C.B., Ninan, P.T., Ballenger, J., Feiger, A., Shrivastava, R.K., Wisselink, P.G., and Wilcox, C.S., Double-blind multicenter comparison of fluvoxamine versus sertraline in the treatment of depressed outpatients. *Depression* 3:163–169, 1995.

13. Feiger, A., Kiev, A., Shrivastava, R.K., *et al.* Nefazodone versus sertraline in outpatients with major depression: Focus on efficacy, tolerability, and effects on sexual function and satisfaction. *Journal of Clinical Psychiatry* 57(Suppl. 2): 53–62, 1996.

14. Preskorn, S.H. Comparison of the tolerability of bupropion, fluoxetine, imipramine, nefazodone, paroxetine, sertraline, and venlafaxine. *Journal of Clinical Psychiatry* 56(Suppl.): 12–21, 1995.

15. Bacon, R. The effects of antidepressants on human sexuality: Diagnosis and management update 1996. *Primary Psychiatry* 4: 32–38, 1997.

16. Shrivastava, R.K., Shrivastava, S., Overweg, N., and Schmitt, M. Amantadine in the treatment of sexual dysfunction associated with selective serotonin reuptake inhibitors (letter to the editor). *Journal of Clinical Psychopharmacology* 15(1): 83–84, 1995

17. Ashton, A.K., Hamer, R., and Rosen, R.C. Serotonin reuptake inhibitor-induced sexual dysfunction and its treatment: A large-scale retrospective study of 596 psychiatric outpatients. *Journal of Sex and Marital Therapy* 23(3): 165–175, 1997.

18. Narder, M.J. Buspirone treatment of sexual dysfunction associated with selective serotonin reuptake inhibitors. *Depression* 2: 109–112, 1995.

19. Arnott, S., and Nutt, D. Successful treatment of fluvoxamine-induced anorgasmia by cyproheptadine. *British Journal of Psychiatry* 164: 838–839, 1994.

20. Kapur, S., Zipursky, R.B., Jones, C., Wilson, A.A., Dasilva, J.D., and Houle, S. Cyproheptadine: A potent in vivo serotonin antagonist (letter to the editor). *American Journal of Psychiatry* 153(6):884, 1997.

21. Bartlik, B.D., Kaplan, P.M., and Kocsis, J.H. 5 psychostimulants apparently reverse sexual dysfunction secondary to selective serotonergic re-uptake inhibitors. *Journal of Sex and Marital Therapy* 21(4):264–271, 1996.

22. Reynolds, R.D. Sertraline-induced anorgasmia treated with intermittent Nefazodone (letter to the editor). *Journal of Clinical Psychiatry* 58(2): 89, 1997.

23. Seagraves, R.T. Treatment of drug-induced anorgasmia (letter to the editor). *British Journal of Psychiatry* 165:554, 1995.

24. Thompson, T.L. (Chair). Management of sexual dysfunction in depression: A continuing medical education symposium at the American Psychiatric Association's 1997 Annual Meeting, San Diego, CA.

25. Goldman, E.L. Ginkgo eases drug-induced sex dysfunction. Report of A.J. Cohen's American Psychiatric Association's 1997 Annual Meeting, San Diego, California. *Clinical Psychiatry News* July 1997, p. 5.

26. Rosenblatt, M., and Mindel, J. Spontaneous hyphema associated with ingestion of *Ginkgo biloba* extract (letter to the editor). *New England Journal of Medicine* 336(15):1108, 1997.

27. Anderson, I., and Tominson, B. Treatment discontinuation with selective serotonin reuptake inhibitors compared with tricyclic antidepressants: A meta-analysis. *British Medical Journal* 310:1433–1438, 1995.

28. Mir, S., and Taylor, D. The adverse effects of antidepressants. *Current Opinion in Psychiatry* 10(2):88–94, 1997.

29. Bancroft, J. *The Pharmacology of Sexual Function and Dysfunction*. Excerpta Medica: Amsterdam, 1995.

30. Pomerantz, S.M. Monoamine influences on male sexual behavior of nonhuman primates. In: J. Bancroft (ed.), *The Pharmacology of Sexual Function and Dysfunction*. Excerpta Medica: Amsterdam, 1995, pp. 201–214.

31. Marsden, C.A. The neuropharmacology of serotonin in the central nervous system. In: J.P. Feighner and W.F. Boyer (eds.), *Selective Serotonin Reuptake Inhibitors* (2nd ed.). Advances in Basic Research and Clinical Practice). Wiley: New York, 1996, p. 23.

32. Bancroft, J. The effects of a new α-2 adrenoreceptor antagonist on sleep and nocturnal penile tumescence in normal male volunteers and men with erectile dysfunction. *Psychosomatic Medicine* 57(4):345–356, 1995.

33. Jacobson, F.M. Fluoxetine-induced sexual dysfunction and an open trial of yohimbine. *Journal of Clinical Psychiatry* 53:119–122, 1992.
34. Gitlin, M.J. Psychotropic medications and their effects on sexual function: Diagnosis, biology, and treatment. *Journal of Clinical Psychiatry* 55(9):406–413, 1994.
35. Hsu, J.H., and Shen, W.W. Male sexual side effects associated with antidepressants: A descriptive clinical study of 32 patients. *International Journal of Psychiatric Medicine* 25:191–201, 1995.
36. Rothchild, A.J. Selective serotonin reuptake inhibitor-induced sexual dysfunctions: Efficacy of a drug holiday. *American Journal of Psychiatry* 152:1514–1516, 1995.
37. Schiavi, R.C., and Segraves, R.T. The biology of sexual function. *Psychiatric Clinics of North America* 18(1):7–24, 1995.
38. Morales, A., Heaton, J.W.P., and Condra, M. The pharmacology of impotence. In A.H. Bennett (ed.), *Impotence: Diagnosis and Management of Erectile Dysfunction*. Saunders: Philadelphia, 1994, pp. 145–155.
39. Rosen, R. Alcohol and drug effects on sexual response: Human experimental and clinical studies. In: J. Bancroft, C.M. Davis, and H.J. Ruppel (eds.), *Annual Review of Sex Research: An Integrative and Interdisciplinary Review*. Society for the Scientific Study of Sex: Lake Mills, IA, 1991, Vol. II, pp. 119–180.

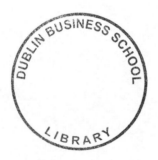

10

On Being a Middle-Aged Therapist

By design and repeated choice, I spend the majority of my work hours with patients. The clinical opportunities and obligations still beckon me, in part because over time I get better at dealing with them, and in part because new problems keep appearing.[1] Early in my career I saw the typical hospital-oriented difficulties that psychiatrists are still called on to deal with—depression, anxiety, psychosis, and substance abuse. I began to specialize in the promising field of clinical sexuality. In doing so, I came to understand in a different way some of the problems brought to general psychiatrists.

AN INFORMAL HISTORY OF CLINICAL SEXUALITY

People with marital discord, sexual dysfunctions, gender identity disorders, struggles with homosexuality, and paraphilia began to ask me for help. Many of them were young adults within 10 years of my age. They educated me. In the middle to late 1970s, sex therapists concentrated on premature ejaculation, psychogenic impotence, female anorgasmia,[2] and gender identity disorders. By the late 1970s, a new wave of patients appeared. People sought help for the absence of sexual desire, and in doing so, taught us that sex therapy techniques were insufficient for people with these dilemmas. By 1980, we had learned that helping people with sexual problems was not simple. Some of the

173

"deeper" psychological constructs that were rejected with the advent of sex therapy seemed necessary once again, particularly after biological investigations failed to explain the low levels of desire. Sex therapists in the 1980s began to appreciate the interpersonal and individual developmental forces that generated and maintained sexual interest. Ideological differences began to be less strident as no professional approach was able to claim consistent success with the loss of desire.

In the late 1970s, society was also beginning to discover the high incidence of childhood sexual abuse. As the data mounted, a new flood of women and men appeared. The women came seeking psychological assistance for their remote childhood sexual abuse; the men—incest offenders, pedophiles, exhibitionists, and voyeurs—came with socially unacceptable sexual behaviors.[3] Excessive sexual desire began to emerge as a separate problem. By the mid-1980s, therapists became more cognizant of compulsive seeking of anonymous partners in parks and pornographic movie houses, and of prostitutes and of partnerless relentless masturbation.

The care of impotent men changed dramatically in 1986 with the introduction of intracavernosal injections. This treatment stimulated a great deal of urological research. Discoveries were made in the basic mechanisms of erection and erectile dysfunction and significant treatment advances materialized. By the early 1990s medical treatment of male sexual woes received another assist from the reports that the newer SSRI antidepressant medications were useful in treating premature ejaculation.

Professional sexual misconduct was discovered in the 1990s. The mental health and medical professions strongly reiterated their ethical positions on sex with current and former patients and clients. As the United States was swept by computer technology advances and more people used the internet, new sexual compulsivities appeared.[4]

THE THERAPIST AS EDUCATOR AND INVESTIGATOR

Even though the forms of sexual problems have evolved, patients with marital discord, sexual dysfunction, gender identity struggles, and

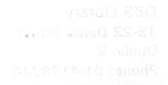

paraphilias still frequently seek assistance. As a result, I get to play two almost distinct roles:

The Educator with the Familiar Problems

I have been taking care of people with sexual dysfunctions for many years and have become so accustomed to their personal stories that I sometimes feel like I can finish my new patients' sentences. I view these patients as my personal challenges to find the right words to demystify their experience, to enable them to face more clearly what created the problem, and to overcome the problem. Their issues quickly engage me as I tell myself, "If you really understand this matter so well, you ought to be able to efficiently help this person!" I educate them about their intrapsychic process; they recognize immediately that I am largely correct, and it changes them in some positive manner. Often their symptoms disappear!

The Investigator with the Less Familiar Problems

Although the patient with a relatively new-to-me problem has engaged me to be a therapist, I initially feel that I am more an investigator in highly unfamilar territory. "What do I know about this subject?" "What is the problem here?" "Did something go wrong with this person's early development?" "Is a definable biological abnormality present?" "Is this simply a very bad choice that this person made?" "What can I do about it?" Eventually, if I come to deeply understand the problem from work with a number of patients, the new problem becomes familiar and I can proceed more efficiently. This has been true with the diverse problems that have always existed in our culture but were not conceptualized in 1975: the dilemmas caused by extramarital affairs; celibates struggling to find happiness through a spiritual life; the ever-changing forms of sexual compulsivities; professional sexual misconduct; the disappearance of all sexual desire after marriage; erotic transference; longstanding father incest, and others. Therapy becomes a joint process whereby the patient and I try to help each other understand and overcome. It is far less efficient, however, than with the seemingly simpler more familiar problems. The results are often far less dramatic.

Personal Identity

This body of clinical experiences has led me to a clearer understanding of how I have interpreted my life as a psychiatrist. My personal rendition of a mental health professional is that my obligation is to stay directly occupied with understanding the pathogenesis of mental distress and the art of its alleviation. This includes attention to the distress of the otherwise reasonably healthy and the mentally ill. My identity as a clinician is based on the self-serving assumption that between the need to better understand what is going on with patients and the ambition to find a way of offering significant assistance, my professional life ought to remain absorbing for a lifetime.

This commitment to stay directly engaged with patients is not the only way of being a psychiatrist. Some of my colleagues are busy administrating, teaching, testifying in lawsuits, or running research grants, hospital divisions, or services in the community. These are different psychiatric careers. I have sampled some of these activities. I have administrated, designed and conducted some research, run the research studies designed in pharmaceutical companies, taught general adult psychiatry to psychiatric residents, psychology fellows, and medical students, given my "expert medical opinion" to lawyers, and held forth on sexuality to anyone who would listen. Even after occasional forays into these activities, I return to my central professional identity. What I like to do most of all, most of the time, is to try to realize my therapeutic ambitions. In a field that is constantly searching for its identity, constantly generating new data and new roles for psychiatrists, this traditional one is simply mine.[5]

Therapeutic Ambitions

Now I consider my therapy work to contain evidence of six clinical ambitions:

1. *It begins with a quest to gain a clear perspective about the social and psychological dilemmas of the patient.* It is not

merely a multiaxial diagnostic exercise. The quest requires a synthesis that I could not achieve when I was younger. The clinical synthesis is important to me because I perceive that much of adult emotional suffering is generated in the processes of creating and solving personal dilemmas. It is important for the patient because the synthesis enables the patient to better understand and realistically deal with the situation. When I provide a tentative synthesis to the patient, my words, metaphors, and examples from the lives of others are carefully chosen to influence.

2. *It is a subtle pursuit of emotional genuineness.* Although much of therapy attempts to focus on defensiveness, dishonesty, and the patient's avoidance of the relevant issues, I prefer to flip these concepts on their opposite surfaces and see them as means of avoiding emotional genuineness. I am actively trying to help the patient to be comfortably genuine with him- or herself. This typically begins by doing everything I can think of to insist that we create an interpersonal honesty between ourselves in therapy.

3. *It is an attempt to diminish suffering through assisting each patient to evolve a new viewpoint about their dilemmas.* The new outlook is based on several conceptual tools that are thoroughly familar to therapists: (a) thoughts are different from behavior; (b) the patient has to learn to identify and comfortably tolerate a fuller range of personal thoughts and emotions; (c) it is the nature of human beings to privately struggle with something; (d) behavior has consequences. Other useful ideas may be less commonly appreciated: (e) one's current feelings are not necessarily the most important matter—other people's views or needs may be more important; (f) struggling with an issue over time facilitates maturation; (g) it may be dangerous to be too certain that this matter is out of your control. This list is not exhaustive, of course, and other ideas must influence what happens as well. But the therapist's concepts often combine to help patients to grow calmer with their internal processes. This calmness is experienced as relief. Even when modest, relief helps the patient and the therapist to realize how changeable some forms of misery are. Hope follows.

4. *It is a search to find a medication that might lighten the distress and burden of the patient.* This process grants considerable respect to the patient's wishes regarding taking medication. It creates a discussion of all objections and requires waiting until the patient has decided to risk the drawbacks for the potential benefits.[6] Many patients who are initially insistent that they do not want to use medication eventually take it to their benefit. Many others who easily accept a trial of medication, find that their use of the drug is short-lived because of either side effects, ineffectiveness, or psychotherapy has helped to solve the problem in another way.

5. *It is an indirect attempt to prevent the recurrence of similar suffering.* I sense myself to be a more active than passive therapist. I want to accurately conceptualize the problem and facilitate some more effective engagement with it so that the person makes progress. Although I am a supportive person, I do not envision my work to be merely supportive. I do not look forward to just being with patients, hearing their anguish, and having them return for years to tell me how terrible their spouse is, for instance. I sometimes joke with a patient who might settle with this type of therapy that the purpose of our visits is not to help me remodel my house. If we do our work well as a team, I am looking to prevent future suffering of the same sort that brought the patient to see me in the first place.

6. *It is an attempt to increase respect for the developmental processes of living.* The concept of pathology may be useful for diagnostic and insurance purposes, but for therapeutic ones, psychopathology usually refers to the suffering that follows the failure to deal effectively with definable issues. An issue may be a discrete past experience or a less defined relationship process or some current developmental task. Ultimately, I am trying to help people to appreciate the individuality of their lives, to respect their past and present, and to clarify how they would like to spend their limited futures. What may have begun with pathology,should give way to enhanced appreciation

of the self and others and of personal potentialities and limitations.

PROFESSIONAL MATURATION

The clarification of these ambitions occurred during my middle age. Therapy has become an easier process for me. Now I am able to tell myself that I have "conversations" with patients. I talk more in sessions. When I was a younger therapist, I proudly, self-righteously, listened more. Back then, I would not have described what I did as "conversation." I would have stressed the importance of the patient talking, of unconscious processes, of the insight that our relationship induced, and of the transference. Not that these factors are unimportant, but I have strengthened my sense of responsibility to actively contribute to the patient's welfare. What the patient thinks, feels about me and our relationship, and does or does not do with our sessions are still the major ingredients, but now I think that I am being paid for something beside listening attentively and nonspecific reflexive support. I am being paid to catalyze improvement. My attentive good listening is only the beginning of my work. The telling of the story is only the beginning of the patient's work. If patients rarely think about the content of our sessions, we probably are wasting our time. Therapy is supposed to engage a person in something deep and personal. Even a disturbing conversation with me is far better than a response that keeps the conversations "interesting" but unprocessed. Therapy may be just conversation but it is a serious, earnest purposeful process.[7]

Since aspiring to be a physician, I have liked the demand for trustworthiness, knowledge, and high-quality one-sided psychological intimacy that are integral to the doctor–patient relationship. My understanding of this relationship has evolved dramatically, however. Research and writing in general adult psychiatry are currently not preoccupied with the primary problems that are brought to me. My clinical experience has dealt with the sexual conundrums of individuals, couples, and society. But their sexual problems, I finally see, are just my patients' ticket into these hopeful conversations. Regardless of the presenting problem, therapeutic relationships require professional skills that are built on a foundation of ethical trustworthiness, knowledge, and high-quality listening and speaking. Although I probably intuitively understood that these demands were essential to professionalism in medical school, in the last decade these matters have been made quite explicit. The pathways to professional sexual misconduct have been well characterized, society has broadly discussed its expectations of teachers, psychotherapists, clergy, and physicians, and I have been privileged to have seen many men and women who have ethically transgressed. Ethical therapy may not significantly help some patients, but grossly unethical behavior, however rationalized by the therapist and patient, holds a potential to greatly harm each of them and their families.[8]

The Emotional Moments of Maturation

The signs of my professional growth have often been heralded by the surprise appearance of embarrassment and exhilaration. These two feelings arose when I became aware that one of my important ideas was likely to be incorrect. I term these defunct ideas my professional illusions. The explosions of these illusions are always shocking. Here are a few ideas that used to constitute what I believed as a younger psychiatrist: Childhood conflicts were the most important source of adult problems; my patients share everything that is relevant with me; the ideas of my esteemed teachers are essentially correct; the therapist should not give advice; my understanding of the patient's situation is relatively complete; being loved is enough to make a person consistently happy, there are two sexes and two genders, I understand the cause of mental symptoms.

Illusions Are Still Present

I think in new ways about my work and I behave differently. My patients are older but still hover around 10 years on either side of my age. I am calmer, less apt to be certain, and occasionally more certain. During therapy I smile, laugh, talk, and use earthy language more than ever before. "Dr. Levine, you are always so serious" is now only rarely thrown at me. My skepticism has increased considerably. I now know that people withhold highly relevant information from me. I better understand why the principle of autonomy occupies the pinnacle in the hierarchy of ethical values that governs medicine. I have lost respect for some of the formulaic ideas that my teachers believed formed the basis of good therapy. I have become privately dismissive of psychiatric ideologies. I now find offensive the self-serving demagogic misinformation about the nature of psychiatric illness—it is a brain disease, it is genetic, it is caused by the mother, it was the sexual abuse, it is a classical oedipal problem—that various elements of our society collude to generate.[9] I am not asserting that I am correct in my perceptions. I am only saying that, along with my profession and the health care environment, I am independently changing. I know that I still have professional illusions because I still have moments of surprise—moments of embarrassment followed by exhilaration when I realize that I am about to learn something important once again.

Middle-Aging

I am aging. My knowledge has not proven as powerful as I thought it might when I was younger. I am far more aware of the limitations of my knowledge than my knowledge per se. I am occasionally reminded by interacting with some patients that there is profound merit to the idea that some people suffer from a brain process that cannot be influenced positively by my brand of conversation, with or without medication. I am often reminded that I am unable to change the profound organizing influence of the patient's past experiences even though this hope brought the patient into therapy. I fervently support the idea, which I cannot personally encompass, that psychiatry must make room for diverse paradigms and approaches.[10] But our education must be broad enough to welcome the relevant issues that are usually discussed by the humanities rather than restricted to more limited conceptions and data productions of clinical science. I know that I do not know how to accomplish this.

Pathogenesis in Mid-Life

In my view, patients do not just have a psychiatric diagnosis, such as major depression, obsessive-compulsive disorder, generalized anxiety disorder, paraphilia, or alcoholism. They have continuous lives characterized by struggles along some developmental line or with a specific developmental task. When they fail to attain a desired goal, they often develop some set of symptoms. Unfortunately, for many middle-aged people this proves to be cumulative: Developmental tasks that were poorly accomplished seem to be compounded by the inability to meet subsequent challenges.

Because psychiatry has largely abandoned sexuality as a topic, it is not surprising that many of my patients have problems that are rarely mentioned in the major psychiatric journals. They have difficulties in the spheres of loving, intimacy, or sexuality that have played an important role in the development of their various comorbidities. The patients of other mental health professionals have similar difficulties, of course. Many of my patients have made decisions that have not turned out well. I perceive this most clearly when I participate in their decision-making processes. They have to make difficult choices regarding relationships about which they often cannot clearly think or cannot readily discuss. This provides important ways to be of help: clear thinking; accurate articulation of the patient's feelings, perceptions, and dilemmas; anticipating consequences; weighing benefits and the risks of every course of action; respect for the complexity inherent in such choices; and patience.

Once therapy begins, what they decide and how they implement their choices often seem more important than their diagnosis. Watching this process, it often spontaneously occurs to both of us that their decompensated state may have been the result of their previous choices. There is a tautology here. Bad decisions create negative consequences, but what produces the tendency to bad decisions? Neurosis? What do we mean by that? Addiction? What are we talking about? Mental illness? Do we mean something other than meeting criteria for a diagnosis? Every answer may have some merit but clinicians should hold themselves to a high standard in seeking a causal explanation for mental suffering. Every answer is merely an invitation to ask, "What do I mean by that?" Hopefully, middle-aged professionals have learned that it is far safer to be engaged in this never-ending search for understanding than to assert such finalities as it is an oedipal problem, an abnormal discharge of the nucleus ceruleus, it is her struggle with her mother, or, the most egregious, it is a chemical imbalance.

Others have said this well. Here is Lipowski on using oversimplifications as explanations:[11]

It confuses the distinction between etiology and correlation, and cause and mechanism, a common confusion in our field. It gives the patient the misleading impression that his or her imbalance is *the* cause of his or her illness, that it needs to be fixed by chemical means, that psychotherapy is useless, and that personal efforts and responsibility have no part to play in getting better.... To assume...that biochemical processes underlie mental activity and behavior does not imply that they are the causal agents but rather constitute mediating mechanisms. They are influenced by the information inputs we receive from our body and environment and by the subjective meaning of that information for us. It is the meaning which largely determines what we think, feel, and do.

Middle-Aged Rewards

I am not entirely certain why many of my patients spontaneously say that they benefit from our conversations, relationship, process, or whatever we call therapy. They often tell me something that I said in a previous session was very helpful. Sometimes I do not even remember uttering the sentence. It, of course, pleases me because it seems that my heart is in the right place and that I might be getting better at the work. Some people emphasize that the therapy was helpful even though the symptom that brought them to therapy did not change. I am sure this is the experience of many of my colleagues as well. People remember our names and our relationships with them. They come to trust us. This is one of the rewards for devoting oneself to the quasi-scientific art of psychiatry, to seeing patients and conceptualizing the role of the mental health professional as one that struggles to relieve and prevent emotional suffering.

Sadly, this reminds me of my younger colleagues who are now seeking jobs rather than careers. Already they are switching from employer to employer without a focus, a theme, that they can explore for years, decades, or a lifetime. They are becoming fungible cogs in a wheel; patients do not remember their names.

Well, it is a different world today, Dr. Levine, nobody believes that psychiatrists should really do therapy—particularly long-term therapy. We are trained to diagnose, evaluate, use pharmacotherapy, and to supervise the care given by less expensively trained professionals.

I lament that the young of our profession are not seeking opportunities to be with patients long enough to understand the processes that shape their lives, that is, that create the psychopathological states about which we claim to have expertise. How emotionally satisfying can this be over a lifetime? What will they have as an antidote for the poisonous continuing thought "I really don't know what I'm doing" that afflicts the young credentialed in every mental health field? You see, I *am* aging: I have become old enough to worry about the young.

THE VALUE OF SURPRISE

Dr. Levine, I told my wife that I would occasionally stop in to see you as a condition of returning to live with her 9 months ago. I thought it was time to see you again. You won't believe what I did after we stopped our monthly meetings. I told my wife I wanted to come back and would end my relationship with the other woman. I broke up with Sherry by writing her a long letter and then I left town for a week. That was after our last visit. She tracked me down by phone in Vegas. She was crying hysterically and telling me all the reasons why I should not end our relationship, just like she had in the past. I agreed with her and agreed to continue to see her. There are so many things that I like about her—she is clean, cooks well, keeps a neat house, is fun to be with, and I feel like I am young again with her, young in a way that I missed when I was her age. But at the very same time that I was intending to become a faithful husband for the first time in 5 years, I started a new sexual relationship with my 32-year-old secretary. We connected because Gloria and I both lost our fathers when we were young. Before I knew it, I was cheating on my wife, cheating on Sherry, and cheating on Gloria. I used to be such a straight arrow. I don't know who I am anymore.

I know that when I left therapy it was clear that I had fixed the situation and was feeling much better. Not only did I not actually do what I intended, I made everything much worse. Monday with my wife, Tuesday with Sherry, and Wednesday with Gloria. I was going crazy fabricating stories. The sex was good—at least with my girlfriends. My wife and I have had sex twice in 9 months; she liked it, I think, but it was pretty tame for me. Sherry and Gloria eventually got together and confronted me. I paid Gloria a large amount of money and she left to work elsewhere. I think my problem is just that I am a liar: I cannot tell the truth to a woman. What is wrong with me?

Indeed, what is wrong with this 49-year-old man who says what he wants to do, works toward the goal with seeming seriousness, and finally refuses —claiming inability—to do what he says? Unconscious ambivalence? Self-deception? Deceit of the therapist? Inadequate therapy? Cowardice? Foolish therapist? All of the above?

When a patient asks me this question, I often can feel myself smiling at its profundity. It makes me aware of how little I know and how wrong the patient is to assume that I can answer it. I am too skeptical and too respectful of the person's membership in the human family to offer an explanation.

One of the values of seeing patients returning to the same therapist is that we have opportunities to see how powerful our therapy proved in reorganizing the patient's approach to life. In cases like the one above, therefore, we have an opportunity to have another professional developmental moment, namely, surprise. This is a constant reminder to stay humble.

REFERENCES

1. Levine, S.B. What is clinical sexuality? *Psychiatric Clinics of North America* 18(1): 1–6, 1995.
2. Masters, W.H., and Johnson, V. *Human Sexual Inadequacy.* Little, Brown: Boston, 1970.
3. Abel, G.G., and Rouleau, J.L. Sexual abuses. *Psychiatric Clinics of North America* 18(1): 139–154, 1995.
4. Cooper, A. Special issue: Sexuality and the internet. *Journal of Sex Education and Therapy* 22(1): 3–91, 1997.

5. Freedman, D.X. The search: Body, mind, and human purpose. *American Journal of Psychiatry* 149(7): 858–866, 1992.
6. Appelbaum, P.S., and Gutheil, T.G. Drug refusal: A study of psychiatric inpatients. *American Journal of Psychiatry* 137: 340–346, 1980.
7. Jackson, S.W. The listening healer in the history of psychological healing. *American Journal of Psychiatry* 149(12): 1623–1632, 1992.
8. Lazarus, J.A. Sex with former patients almost always unethical (editorial). *American Journal of Psychiatry* 149(7): 855–857, 1992.
9. Eisenberg, L. The social construction of the human brain. *American Journal of Psychiatry* 152(11): 1563–1575, 1995.
10. Gabbard, G.O. Psychodynamic psychiatry in the "decade of the brain." *American Journal of Psychiatry* 149(8): 991–998, 1992.
11. Lipowski, Z.J. Psychiatry: Mindless or brainless, both or neither? *Canadian Journal of Psychiatry* 34: 249–254, 1989.

11

One Avenue to Spiritual Love

O love is the crooked thing,
There is nobody wise enough,
To find out all that is in it.
—W.B. Yeats, from *Brown Penny*

IS DEATH THE MOTHER OF BEAUTY?

As many people move into their middle years, they become sensitive to the strong bias toward youth in many cultural arenas. This discovery is typically associated with a feeling of being excluded from membership in a seemingly elite category. Of course, there are many ways of coping with this inevitability, but humor is probably among the best. In fact, many in the over-40 group can be overheard talking about the discovery of their youthful illusions. They may lightheartedly refer to their previous assumptions that they possessed permanence, a guarantee of a future, an invulnerability from accident and disease, or an easy access to sexual pleasure. By the middle years, such notions are clearly unfounded. The embarrassment of once having held them gives rise to self-mockery about one's foolishness.

The middle-aged have learned that youthful potentialities are just that and that they, and many others, have failed to realize their opportunities. This is not mere idle psychological process, however; it is a preparation for appreciating the present and the future. Loss of youthful potential helps people to conduct their lives more seriously, to be more realistic about their ambitions, and act as though they do not have forever to attain them. Many middle-aged people know that health,

187

opportunity, and life itself are not forever. Personal tragedy—that is, premature serious illness, accident, and death—are distinct possibilities.

Wallace Stevens succinctly captured this phenomenon with the line, "Death is the mother of beauty" in his poem *Sunday Morning*. It is not just death, however, that holds the potential to create a new aesthetic appreciation. Less complete losses—including lost opportunities—can propel us into a greater awareness of oneself, of the partner, of friends, of children, of nature, and of the other elements of one's life that are now valued. Because nothing is actually permanent, an imperative arises to find and appreciate the beauty of the transient.

AS LONG AS THERE IS LIFE LOVE CAN GROW

The aesthetics of loss contribute to the sex and love dramas of the middle-aged. Sex and love are not the same as they were initially experienced in phases 2 (establishment of the sexual equilibrium), 3 (preservation of sexual behavior), or 4 (physiological declines of the 50s). Nonetheless, these dramas continue to generate the potential for pleasure or despair during and after the middle years.

This chapter is concerned with a potential love drama of powerful proportion that exists within phase 6 (the arrival of serious illness) of some couples. For them, phase 6 is not just adversity, it is also a developmental phase, an opportunity. The developmental potential of illness is far from universal. Not all illnesses create the possibility of deepening love; many are just tests of the capacity to abide the decline of the partner and do the right thing by well caring for the partner. To fully realize the developmental potential of love that is inherent in serious illness, the sick person's mental capacities must be modestly intact.

Any illness that reduces the person to weakness, vulnerability, and helplessness can generate it. The illness can be temporary, permanent, or fatal. The person with the illness may be young, middle-aged, or older. What is essential is that the relatively healthy partner have an inescapable evidence that the body is not forever, life can end, health is a precious possession and cannot be taken for granted, and that *this is really happening to both of us*. Illness can be awesome and the partner must witness its power and sense the awe.

DISCOVERY OF SPIRITUAL LOVE

Successful outcomes of this era's developmental challenge can be alternatively stated:

- It can provide a deeper sense of loving the partner.
- It is an opportunity to learn more about oneself in love.
- It is a chance to understand love in a new way.
- It is an occasion to appreciate the partner in a new way that makes the most of the difficulties of the past seem relatively unimportant.
- It demonstrates the cycle of life.
- It can emotionally introduce the person to love's spiritual dimension.

The discovery of spiritual love is not merely a religious experience, a finding of God, or a dedication to a new set of rules given by an organized religion. Atheists can discover spiritual love through illness. Religious feelings may be triggered by spiritual love but they are not necessary to the experience. The stimulus to the realization of a dimension of love that is called spiritual in this culture is an honest empathic encounter with the new realities of the physically ill partner.

The larger social challenge for the healthy person is to provide personal care, private or intrapsychic caring, and valued companionship to the sick person. Obviously, this is a difficult task. Caring for the sick readily becomes a burden. It fills us with fatigue, confronts us with our sense of obligation, makes us remember our past disappointments, challenges us to abandon our own needs, and exposes us to our anger over *our* fate. We humans—even those of us who are physicians—are generally afraid of illness, of decline, and of death. We often find subtle ways to avoid situations with our families and friends when serious illness strikes. A card, a brief occasional visit, or a get well gift-will suffice—we hope. But, eventually, we are confronted: It is our parent, spouse, or child. It is our developmental task to be there, to care, to comfort, to overcome our narcissism—we either rise to the occasion to a sufficient degree or we do not.

The illness experience in a partner is not the only avenue to spiritual love. When a partner's body is diminished by illness, the deepening appreciation of loving the partner is not simply a transient mental relief from the social burdens of illness. It is a comfort to the healthy one. It is the opportunity to create a capstone for the life shared: "We do love each other. It does not depend on sex, status, money, friends, travel, golf. The matters that used to bother me about you are now unimportant. What is important is that we connect in this basic elemental caregiving way." As long as this juxtaposition exists—two relatively intact minds, one relatively intact body, and one failing body—love can continue to grow.

What enables the experience of spiritual love to be recognized as something distinctly beyond the previous sensations of love is the heightened appreciation of the partner, the self, and the link to the natural universe and its inherent cycles of birth, life, and death. The partner's beauty, dignity, individuality, and frailty are seen not just as characteristics of the person, but as characteristics shared by all people. One is part of the cosmos, the universe, something unfathomably large—larger than ever before appreciated in quite this way. The discovery of a larger more intense love, a more powerful beauty, at a time when the body of the person has few of the traits that one previously found sexually attractive is not only a relief but a life changing experience. A person often feels that he or she finally understands this love thing. It is sensed as vitally important—a pinnacle experience. It is spiritual.

SPIRITUAL APPRECIATION OF LOVE IS TRANSIENT AND CAN RECUR AFTER DEATH

Although the realization of this kind of love is a profoundly satisfying experience that reorders the healthy partner's perceptions, feelings, and capacities to abide, it often does not last. The burden of caring for the ill is often too great. The sick partner's mind often slips, his or her behavior regresses, and the physical losses further intensify. The process become an ordeal that must be endured. When death does occur, love for the partner often is reintensified and sensed again as spiritual. This time, however, the absence of the partner creates a whole new set of circumstances that require accommodation. Mentally, that is, privately, love for the partner can reach its purest, most perfect form when the actual burdens of providing care and watching the decline are over. The aggressive impurities of love for the partner are often removed by some psychological process; the memories, feelings about, and meanings of the previous relationship either improve on the past realities or come to be appreciated in a new way that enables a more fixed intense love of the deceased.

Vignette One: Finally Getting There

The affair has been over for 3 years. He occasionally sees the younger woman, who is now his friend, during sexless visits to her home. He is back living full time with his wife who long endured the indignity of her husband's refusal to stop the affair, their friends' knowledge of his carryings-on, and his because this is what I chose to do manner. She got a little psychiatric support and an SSRI from me to keep herself from "jumping out the window."

Her familial tremor, which appeared at age 50, progressively worsened and at age 57 was declared to be Parkinson's disease. Two years of further decline ensued, despite the appropriate medications. Now, her balance is terrible, her energy is markedly lessened, her movements stiffer, and walking has become an ever-uncertain challenge.

But she gets up daily, tends to her routines, and finds the pets and the squirrels, birds, and trees as charming and beautiful as ever. She is grateful for the sunshine. She secludes herself from most acquaintances now, but remains interested in hearing her husband's stories about them. She tries to read but jokes that she has trouble remembering what she just read. Besides an occasional comment on her diminishing capacity, she does not complain much. She seems pleased that he is home, the affair is over, and she has more time with her husband than she has had in years. She has realized her goal of not being abandoned. "Thank God!"

He is no longer angry at her for his sins. He sees her more clearly now—her physical weakness and her tenacious fight to maintain her dignity. For the first time in his life with two wives, he clears the dishes from the table and takes over finishing up in the kitchen because she has no more than 5 minutes of energy at the sink. "I never thought it was my responsibility." He makes *her* lunch now and for the first time, he comes home quickly after work to see how she is.

I ask this highly intellectualized man what all this has been like for him. I remember our past conjoint marital sessions dealing with his affair when he yelled in red-faced anger, squirmed from his barely acknowledged guilt, and stammered over his duplicity, but never do I remember him crying. Now here it is: this previously stone-faced man overcome with sadness, the tears leaking over his handsome face. Suddenly the irony of his chief complaint hits me. He said that when he sat down at this his first visit to me in a year "something feels like it is pulling my lips down into a frown all the time, " After he cries for a few moments, he is able to speak.

Despite her weakness, she is beautiful. I love her. It is so sad to see her like she is.

You mean trapped in her shaking prison.

Yes, but she keeps on. I want to care for her. I am caring for her. There is something sweet about this sadness. What I don't really understand is that I feel love for everything, I feel like I understand things, yet I don't understand what is going on.

Well, you have gained something important. You see her vulnerability, you want to protect her. You see her struggling to maintain her psychological sameness and you wonder if you could have such dignity in the face of your decline.

I know I love her now and I think that she knows I love her. I still say that I love her just like I used to, but I think she knows it now. She smiles at me sometimes in a way I just can't describe except to say it feels good. You know I've spent so much time reading psychology books about love and looking for it. I think I have found it. [He cries again.]

It is nice to see you cry. I wonder whether that sense that your face is pulled down into a perpetual frown is really the consequence of your not permitting yourself any direct expression of your newly discovered intense love for her and the great sadness to finally love deeply a person who is facing a bleak future. Pretty grim, but as you said, there is something beautiful going on here.

Can we talk again?

Sure. [At the next visit, he reported that his facial tightness immediately disappeared and did not return.]

Perhaps most of us need the threat of loss or the witness of a progressive decline to death to come to grips with the intensity of our connection. We who generally value our individuality more highly than our bonds to others must have strong defenses against realizing how deeply attached we are to our partners. Many only discover this on separation, after divorce, or in the weeks and months after a partner's death. It is far easier to intellectually appreciate the idea of a deep connection to a partner, than to permit oneself to feel it. The key question is, "Can we emotionally appreciate the power of our attachments without going through such agonies?"

The answer may be quite disappointing. We have defenses that keep us from being deeply emotionally aroused by love and these may take over quickly once the threat of loss seems to be past.

These periods of intense affective stimulation can and should permanently change us. We should recover from them with the realization that we do cherish our partners, despite their limitations. However nice it is that the stone-faced man finally could realize how much he loved his wife, it is not particularly comforting that it took him to age 60 and required such dire straits to find and activate his simple less narcissistic giving self. At whatever stage it occurs, love remains an exhilarating experience, even when it is admixed with profound sadness.

Vignette Two: Love and Death

Now he is definitely dying. His suffering is controlled by a steady stream of morphine, but the price for his respite is that he is mostly asleep at the hospice, awakening only for a few morsels of food several times a day.

His wife has dealt with his illness admirably. In-home hospice care lasted until he repeatedly pleaded for more relief tearfully saying, "This is no life." Her children, friends, and siblings thought that his transfer from the home would enable her to finally get more sleep, but she remained relatively sleepless away from him. Her days, "beyond fatigue," continued to be spent at his side.

I was privileged to hear about some of this after her husband's last days. Her fear of death had not made a big impression on me during our past work together. Now she reports that her terror of being around a dead person began in the second grade when she had to visit the home of a classmate whose mother had died and was being displayed in the living room. All of the children seemed to know to kneel at the casket and make a sign of the cross. She was terrified about being so close to a dead body, she dissociated and had recurrent nightmares about the experience. She hated horror movies and any thought of death since this experience. Then at age 28, while she was hospitalized with gallbladder colic, she learned that the woman in the next bed had died. "I lost it, became hysterical, and had to be sedated."

At age 57, sitting next to her sleeping husband and often reviewing her life, she is calmly aware that someone dies in the hospice almost everyday. She is no longer intensely fearful. Being with him during these 6 months of decline has inconspicuously resulted in this shift. When death quietly arrived, she was alone with him. After feeling a brief sense of shock and seconds of panic, she quietly got on the bed beside him. She cried silently, peacefully, and repeated, "Goodbye" and "I love you" and "I have always loved you." The staff was unaware of his death for about 20 minutes. Quickly thereafter, the family appeared. She now treasures those final moments with him. "It was spiritual. I was one with him yet separate. I understood. I felt part of the universe."

LOVE AND THE MENTAL HEALTH PROFESSIONAL

Although the middle-aged may transiently long for the pleasures and opportunities of youth or feel offended by their increasing invisibility to the young, these are just minor aspects of our dawning awareness of our personal evolution through the life cycle. Mental health professionals, specialists in the array of emotional decompensations to which humans are susceptible, cannot with impunity turn a blind eye to the processes of life that lead to the decompensations. Of the many lines of development, of the many demands for personal accomplishment that every human being faces, of the numerous ambitions that transiently take hold of our being, those that we call love are most inextricably linked to our essence. What will become of our field if we continue to be professionally disinterested in love?

Index

197

Lightning Source UK Ltd.
Milton Keynes UK
UKOW040611180412

190954UK00001B/2/A

9 780306 484469